Implementing
Evidence-Based Practices
in Behavorial Health

■ ■ ■

Implementing Evidence-Based Practices in Behavorial Health

■ ■ ■

Mark McGovern, Ph.D.

Gregory J. McHugo, Ph.D.

Robert E. Drake, M.D., Ph.D.

Gary R. Bond, Ph.D.

Matthew R. Merrens, Ph.D.

Dartmouth PRC | HAZELDEN®
Evidence-Based Resources for Behavioral Health

Hazelden
Center City, Minnesota 55012
hazelden.org

© 2013 by Dartmouth
All rights reserved. Published 2013.
Printed in the United States of America

Unless a statement on the page grants permission, no part of this publication may be reproduced, stored in a retrieval system, or transmitted in any form or by any means—electronic, mechanical, photocopying, recording, scanning, or otherwise—without the express written permission of the publisher. Failure to comply with these terms may expose you to legal action and damages for copyright infringement.

ISBN: 978-1-61649-458-2

EDITOR'S NOTE

With the exception of the agency director interview, the case examples in this book are drawn from composite examples based on the authors' own professional experiences. The names and details have been changed to protect the privacy of the people involved.

Some minor grammatical or wording changes have been made in the agency director interview transcript and the version of the ACT Fidelity Scale that appears in this book for accuracy.

This publication is not intended as a substitute for the advice of health care professionals.

Alcoholics Anonymous and AA are registered trademarks of Alcoholics Anonymous World Services, Inc.

The Supported Employment Fidelity Scale in this book appears with permission from Dartmouth ©2008, 2011. The Illness Management and Recovery and Assertive Community Treatment fidelity scales appear courtesy of the Substance Abuse and Mental Health Services Administration (SAMHSA).

The implementation measurement tools and fidelity scales on the CD-ROM appear with permission from the following people and organizations. They may be used with the proper acknowledgments:

The Supported Employment Fidelity Scale (2008/2011) and the Agency Readiness for IPS Supported Employment Checklist appear with permission from the Dartmouth Psychiatric Research Center; the Dartmouth Sustainability Interview appears with permission from Gary Bond et al., Dartmouth Psychiatric Research Center; the Dual Diagnosis Capability in Health Care Settings appears with permission from Mark McGovern et al., Dartmouth Psychiatric Research Center; the Assertive Community Treatment Fidelity Scale and Protocol (also known as the Dartmouth Assertive Community Treatment Fidelity Scale and Protocol), the IDDT Fidelity Scale and Protocol, the Family Psychoeducation Fidelity Scale and Protocol, the Illness Management and Recovery Fidelity Scale and Protocol, the General Organizational Index, the Dual Diagnosis Capability in Addiction Treatment, the Dual Diagnosis Capability in Mental Health Treatment, and the MedTEAM Fidelity Scale, Chart, and Protocol appear courtesy of the Substance Abuse and Mental Health Services Administration; the IMR Treatment Integrity Scale, 2011, appears with permission from Alan Benjamin McGuire, Indiana University Purdue University at Indianapolis; the State Health Authority Yardstick (SHAY) Rating Scale, 2007, appears courtesy of the Office of Mental Health, State of New York; the Tool for Measurement of Assertive Community Treatment Summary Scale, 2012, appears with permission from Maria Monroe-DeVita, Lorna Moser, and Gregory Teague.

Cover design: David Spohn
Interior design and typesetting: Kinne Design
Developmental editor: Catherine Creswell

Dartmouth PRC
Hazelden

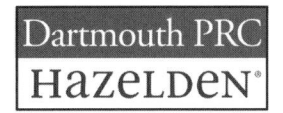

The Dartmouth PRC–Hazelden imprint was formed as a partnership between the Dartmouth Psychiatric Research Center (PRC) and Hazelden Publishing, a division of the Hazelden Foundation—nonprofit leaders in the research and development of evidence-based resources for behavioral health.

Our mission is to create and publish a comprehensive, state-of-the-art line of professional resources—including curricula, books, multimedia tools, and staff-development training materials—to serve professionals treating people with mental health, addiction, and co-occurring disorders at every point along the continuum of care.

For more information about Dartmouth PRC–Hazelden and our collection of professional products, visit the Hazelden Behavioral Health Evolution website at www.bhevolution.org.

Contents

About the Authors	ix
Introduction	xi
1 ▪ Stages of Implementation	1
2 ▪ Implementation Measures	29
3 ▪ The Checklist Approach to Implementation: Who Needs to Do What When	51
4 ▪ Implementing Multiple Evidence-Based Practices Simultaneously	73
5 ▪ Conclusion	85
Frequently Asked Questions	89
Interview with an Agency Director	97
Appendix: Implementation Resources	111
Implementing Evidence-Based Practices: An Agency's Tasks, 113	
Supported Employment Fidelity Scale, 117	
Supported Employment Fidelity Scale Score Sheet, 143	
ACT Fidelity Scale and GOI Cover Sheet, 145	
ACT Fidelity Scale, 147	
ACT Fidelity Score Sheet, 153	
Illness Management and Recovery Fidelity Scale, 155	
Illness Management and Recovery Fidelity Scale Score Sheet, 160	
Contents of the CD-ROM	161
References	163
Recommended Reading and Resources	167

About the Authors

Mark McGovern, Ph.D., is a professor of Psychiatry and of Community and Family Medicine at Dartmouth Medical School and a faculty member of the Dartmouth Psychiatric Research Center. He received a career development award from the National Institute on Drug Abuse for implementing evidence-based therapies for persons with co-occurring disorders into community addiction treatment settings. His research portfolio has two primary components: (1) evaluation of integrated behavioral therapies for co-occurring disorders and (2) evaluation of benchmark measures for integrated program services in addiction, mental health, and primary care settings. He is also editor in chief of the *Journal of Substance Abuse Treatment*.

Gregory J. McHugo, Ph.D., is research professor of Community and Family Medicine and of Psychiatry at Dartmouth Medical School and at the Dartmouth Psychiatric Research Center. He is an experimental psychologist and evaluation methodologist and has been involved in design, implementation, and analysis of large-scale, randomized controlled trials to evaluate treatment and rehabilitation programs for people with severe mental illness. In partnership with Bob Drake, McHugo has conducted studies on integrated dual disorders treatment, supported employment, homelessness and supported housing, and trauma among people with severe mental illness. He was the chief methodologist for the National Implementing Evidence-Based Practices Project, which studied the implementation of five evidence-based practices for people with severe mental illness in over fifty community mental health centers in eight states. McHugo and Drake are now involved in a long-term project to develop electronic decision supports for mental health clients and practitioners.

Robert E. Drake, M.D., Ph.D., is professor of Psychiatry and of Community and Family Medicine at Dartmouth Medical School and the director of the Dartmouth Psychiatric Research Center. He works actively as a community mental health doctor and supervisor on mental health services research. His research focuses on people with serious mental illnesses and services that help their recovery. Current projects include developing and studying electronic decision support systems to enhance communications and shared decision making between clients and clinicians.

He is also conducting randomized controlled trials of services for clients with first psychotic episodes and for clients with co-occurring substance use.

Gary R. Bond, Ph.D., is professor of Psychiatry at Dartmouth Medical School and at the Dartmouth Psychiatric Research Center. He has collaborated and consulted with mental health centers and policy planners at the state and federal levels on implementation issues for over three decades. He helped develop and evaluate several fidelity measures for evidence-based practices and has authored a handbook for developing fidelity scales. He was an investigator on the National Implementing Evidence-Based Practices Project and has recently begun studying sustainability of evidence-based practices. His research has included numerous multi-site studies on supported employment and assertive community treatment.

Matthew R. Merrens, Ph.D., is adjunct professor of Psychiatry at Dartmouth Medical School and at the Dartmouth Psychiatric Research Center. He has authored textbooks in general, social, personality, and developmental psychology. He has worked in mental health settings as a clinical psychologist. While at the Psychiatric Research Center, he has written many publications including books, manuals, articles, videos, and web pages. In addition, he has developed training courses in evidence-based process in mental health and a distance-learning course in co-occurring disorders.

Introduction

OVER THE PAST DECADE, a considerable amount of attention has been paid to the use of evidence-based practices in behavioral health care. Training programs in medicine, psychology, and counseling have begun to emphasize the value of research-based treatment strategies as the best means for improving health outcomes. The evidence-based practices movement has emerged alongside efforts to provide shared decision making and client access to medical records. These efforts together have gone a long way toward providing the behavioral health care that promotes the most favorable outcomes.

Through our work at the Dartmouth Psychiatric Research Center, we, the authors of this book, have evaluated practice effectiveness in real-world settings and provided consultation and training to providers in the health services system. Over the past twenty-five years we have developed evidence-based practices, created scales and assessment measures, and promoted the best strategies for transitioning these evidence-based practices into usual, customary care.

Our group at Dartmouth has worked to establish psychosocial services for people with serious mental illnesses and stressed the importance of integrated care. The integrated dual disorders treatment (IDDT) program is one such program we developed. IDDT emphasizes the integration of services for people with substance use and mental health disorders. Such co-occurring disorders are not isolated or rare problems. Studies suggest that approximately 50 percent of people diagnosed with mental health disorders also have substance use disorders (Fox et al. 2010, p. 1). Research also indicates that non-integrated and parallel treatment approaches do not provide effective services for this group. Nevertheless, many treatment providers are still not able to provide fully integrated services from one treatment team at one location.

The problem is not that practitioners lack effective treatment strategies. In fact, toolkits for IDDT and other evidence-based practices have been available for nearly ten years. Instead, the problem is that well-documented evidence-based treatments are not commonly made available to clients. One study of clients in two different state mental health systems found that fewer than 10 percent of clients were enrolled in evidence-based psychosocial interventions. In fact, the study's authors noted, "Family psychoeducation, an evidence-based practice, is rarely available and evidence-based supported employment is made available to fewer than 5% of patients" (Lehman and Steinwachs 1998). Effective treatments have been developed, but they are not readily available in the usual health-service settings.

The 2003 findings of the President's New Freedom Commission on Mental Health, unfortunately, in large part remain true today:

> An array of evidence-based medications and psychosocial interventions—typically used together—now allows successful treatment of most mental disorders. Despite these advances in science, many Americans are not benefiting from these investments. Far too often, treatments and services based on rigorous clinical research languish for years rather than being used effectively at the earliest opportunity. (President's New Freedom Commission on Mental Health 2003)

Developing evidence-based behavioral health practices is clearly important, but this alone will not improve health care services. As the Institute of Medicine (2001) notes, the time between developing an effective treatment strategy and incorporating it in typical clinical practice is long—up to fifteen to twenty years. If a practice is widely known, too often it is inconsistently or ineffectively employed (Institute of Medicine 2001). The missing link for getting practices from research into routine health care is effective implementation.

In this book, we will discuss the implementation of evidence-based practices in behavioral health and offer practical strategies for bringing these practices into routine clinical settings. We will look at implementation as a specific process, a set of activities and responsibilities designed to successfully launch a practice and integrate it into routine care.

We know that changes in health care do not come about easily. Examining the history of a relatively simple health care practice—hand washing—can be revealing. You might think that hand washing would be a straightforward practice that is well embedded in health services, but let's look further.

> In another example of delayed implementation, Boston surgeon Atul Gawande (2012) points to the slow dissemination of the recommended treatment for severe migraines. Published guidelines indicate that preventive medication can significantly reduce the frequency of severe migraines; however, as Gawande and the authors of the guidelines note, although these measures were recommended more than ten years ago, over two-thirds of migraine patients still are not receiving this treatment. Gawande also notes similar delays in the treatment of cardiac events. Even though evidence suggests that beta-blockers increase patients' chances of survival after cardiac events, only 50 percent of patients receive them, and it has taken fifteen years to reach that level of dissemination.

Implementing Hand Washing

In 1847, Hungarian physician Ignaz Semmelweis demonstrated that puerperal fever (also known as "childbed fever") was contagious and that its incidence could be drastically reduced by enforcing appropriate hand-washing behavior among medical caregivers. His discovery was met with a cold and hostile response from other physicians. Finding his claim to be contrary to the scientific opinion of the times, Semmelweis's medical colleagues argued that, even if Semmelweis were correct, washing one's hands each time before treating a patient would be too much work. (The doctors, apparently, were not eager to admit that they had caused so many deaths.) It was only after the germ theory of disease became accepted in the late nineteenth century that hand washing was taken seriously as a health care practice.

However, this is not the end of the story. Even though hand washing is accepted as a positive and important health care procedure, its usage is less than optimal. The authors of a 2011 article on hand hygiene in the *New England Journal of Medicine* reported that "health-care associated infections are a threat to patient safety":

> Approximately 5 to 10% of hospitalized patients in the developed world acquire such infections, and the burden of disease is even higher in developing countries. Proper use of hand hygiene is critical to the prevention of these infections, but compliance among health care workers is most often below 40%. (Longtin et al. 2011)

Semmelweis demonstrated the effectiveness of hand washing more than 165 years ago, and here we are—still trying to make it part of standard practice. Even more remarkable is that hand washing may protect the worker from infection and thus is in the practitioner's self-interest. So we are left with a situation in which a relatively simple procedure known to be effective is only marginally implemented.

This is all the more striking because hand washing is a rather simple, straightforward practice. The services that need to be implemented in behavioral health care interventions are certainly more complex and demand that practitioners consider the process of implementation seriously in order to be successful.

The Failure to Implement in Behavioral Health

In order to provide the best services for clients, the mental health system needs to respond to scientific findings and move evidence-based practices into treatment centers in an efficient and prompt manner. However, not unlike hand washing, behavioral health practices supported by research findings have moved slowly and often incompletely into general practice. Studies indicate that it takes an average of seventeen years to turn a mere 14 percent of original research findings into benefit for clients and almost two decades to move 14 percent into general practice. This means that 86 percent of findings never make the transition (Green et al. 2009; Balas and Boren 2000).

Again, it is important to note that just because significant research findings have emerged, it doesn't mean that clinical practice will soon change. Behavioral health centers are complex and fragmented organizations faced with many cost and regulatory pressures. They are challenging settings in which to implement change. In addition, each year practitioners are inundated with thousands of articles containing overwhelming amounts of new information, some of which may have ambiguous or contradictory implications for treatment.

Effective implementation requires thoughtful and proven implementation strategies, strategies that must be carried out across many levels of an organization and at various stages of the implementation process. That is, implementation is synonymous with coordinated change at the organizational or agency level, at the specific program level (such as is the case with programs addressing adult severe mental illnesses), and at the level of individual, clinician practice. It is a process that takes place over phases, beginning with pre-implementation planning and continuing through practice initiation to maintenance. The purpose of this book is to present a practical, straightforward guide to the specific tasks and stages of implementing an evidence-based practice. It is our hope that this guidance will allow readers to more effectively incorporate evidence-based practices into their work and to succeed in providing the best services to their clients.

What's Ahead?

Our book will give the reader an informative, easy-to-use guide to implementing an evidence-based practice. Chapter 1 focuses on the stages of implementation. We describe the basic activities, including the strategies to facilitate the process, as well as common barriers to success. As you will see, effective preparation, implementation, and maintenance are all critical to the overall success of the implemented practice. Chapter 2 describes the process of assessing the implementation, a critical factor in supporting and achieving a successfully employed practice. We identify a number of measures for use with specific evidence-based practices and stress a simplified, pragmatic approach to measurement.

Chapter 3 takes a "checklist approach" to the tasks of implementation. We review the roles of the leaders, administrators, and practitioners involved and the tasks necessary for success. The checklist approach has proved its value in industry and medicine, and we believe that it has utility in implementing change in behavioral health practices.

Chapter 4 illustrates how four related and interlocking clinical skills—motivational interviewing, psychoeducation, cognitive-behavioral interventions, and community-integration interventions—can work as building blocks for implementing complex, agency-wide evidence-based practices for people with serious mental illnesses. Agencies whose clinicians can acquire proficiency in these fundamental clinical skills will find it easier to simultaneously implement the many evidence-based practices they need. This chapter also focuses on the critical roles that administrators and clinical leaders play in the implementation process.

Finally, we offer answers to frequently asked questions, an interview with an agency director in the field, and an appendix with tools, assessments, and other resources to smooth the process of implementation.

1

Stages of Implementation

IMPLEMENTATION OF an evidence-based practice (EBP) unfolds over time. People don't work the way they always have on one day and return the next day to work in a new way. You can replace the furniture or rename the agency overnight, but you can't change the way clinicians practice that quickly or easily. Although this seems obvious, all those involved in the implementation of a new practice must have realistic expectations as to how long the implementation will take and how the process will proceed.

This chapter describes the stages of implementation, as we understand them after having conducted the National Implementing Evidence-Based Practices Project. In this project, investigators from the Dartmouth Psychiatric Research Center and representatives from eight states studied the implementation of five psychosocial interventions for people with serious mental illness. The five evidence-based practices were assertive community treatment (ACT), individual placement and support (IPS) or supported employment, integrated dual disorders treatment (IDDT), family psychoeducation, and illness management and recovery (IMR).

Fifty-three sites across the eight states, predominantly community mental health agencies, implemented one of these practices with the assistance of a state-provided consultant/trainer and a toolkit of written and video materials. Implementation monitors visited the sites each month for two years to observe the activities of agency leaders, clinical supervisors, and frontline clinicians and to describe the implementation through field notes and semi-annual interviews. Fidelity to the EBP model and general organizational characteristics were assessed at six-month intervals throughout the two years of implementation. (Fidelity scales assess adherence to the principles and components of a specific evidence-based practice. Organizational characteristics refer to the core features of a setting that facilitate implementation of any evidence-based practice, such as screening and assessment, outcome monitoring, clinical supervision, and staff training. These assessments are discussed in chapter 2.)

While preparing for the project, we developed a classification system for the activities of implementation. Using this system, implementation monitors assigned each activity they observed and responses to interview questions to one of twenty-six categories called implementation dimensions. The five evidence-based practices differed in many ways, including the changes in agency structure, staffing, and clinical skill acquisition each required. Nevertheless, we found that the twenty-six dimensions encompassed nearly all implementation activities, and this framework provides the basis for the implementation advice in this chapter. Furthermore, despite the differences among the five evidence-based practices, common themes emerged concerning the stages of implementation and the activities that characterize each.

> We propose three primary stages of implementation: preparation, implementation, and maintenance.

Based on our experience in the National Implementing Evidence-Based Practices Project, we propose three primary stages of implementation: preparation, implementation, and maintenance. Preparation is the period when a facility is getting ready to change. Implementation marks the time when people are making the changes required by the new practice. Maintenance reflects the efforts at keeping the practice going once it has been implemented.

No simple formula is available to help us determine how long it will take for a facility to prepare for and implement a new practice. It depends on the context into which the new practice is embedded and on the complexity of the practice itself. As a general rule, however, preparation for a new practice takes six months, and implementation takes one year. Maintenance, of course, lasts indefinitely. We found that well-prepared sites could implement an evidence-based practice with high fidelity to the model in six months, whereas less-prepared sites took longer, and some did not achieve high fidelity by the end of two years. Importantly, some sites were able to implement all five practices with high fidelity by the end of a year. So, although the five practices differ, these differences do not serve to indicate the time needed to reach a high-fidelity implementation. What matters more is the process of implementation and organizational change; that is, the activities of the people responsible for the implementation determine how well and how quickly an evidence-based practice can be effectively employed.

Another key insight to remember: the activities within a stage are not unique to that stage. Activities required when preparing to implement a practice are also activities required in the implementation and maintenance stages. Likewise, the activities carried out in order to implement an evidence-based practice will be required throughout the maintenance phase too. New activities get added at each stage, but those begun in a preceding stage will continue.

It is also important to recognize that changes occur on two major levels, the clinical level and the organizational level. Life would be much simpler if implementation of a behavioral health evidence-based practice was just a matter of supervisors and practitioners acquiring new knowledge and skills. But every implementation requires changes at the organizational level as well, and these are often the most challenging.

To facilitate understanding and to align with the stages of implementation, we grouped the twenty-six dimensions into five domains of activity: prioritization, leadership, workforce, workflow, and reinforcement. Each of these domains contains a range of specific responsibilities and activities. In the pages that follow, we'll describe each domain and how the activities of each help lead to a successful implementation. The full list of the twenty-six dimensions can be found in the appendix and on the CD-ROM (see Implementing Evidence-Based Practices: An Agency's Tasks).

There are many paths to successful implementation of an evidence-based practice. The path described here is somewhat idealized. Your path may differ in many ways for a variety of reasons, but, in one way or another, you will still go through the stages of implementation.

Preparation Stage

Adequate preparation in implementing a new practice is critical. The more time and effort devoted to preparing to implement a practice, the more likely it will succeed. Preparation involves anticipating changes required at both the clinical and organizational levels. It lays the groundwork for implementing the practice. Problems are anticipated, and solutions are developed. Not all barriers to implementation will be anticipated, so part of preparation is developing procedures for handling problems as they arise.

In the ideal case, the first step in the preparation stage involves self-assessment. The following questions should be asked: Why are we making this change? Was this change mandated, and if so, by what

Adequate preparation in implementing a new practice is critical.

authority? What need will the new practice meet? Is our organization able to take on a new practice at this time? Do we have the human and material resources to implement the practice? This kind of self-assessment is necessary in order to be realistic about the prospects for successfully implementing a new practice.

After conducting a thoughtful and thorough assessment, the organization then confronts the *decision* whether or not to adopt the practice, and new questions arise. Okay, so we think that we want to adopt the new practice, but is this the time to do it? Do we have sufficient commitment from the top to the bottom levels of our organization to make the implementation happen? Is the larger context supportive of this change? That is, is the mental health authority behind it, is the community ready for it, and are clients and their families prepared for it? To explore this stage of the implementation process further, let's consider a case example.

The Lonesome Dove Agency

The executive director of the Lonesome Dove Agency, a large mental health center, wanted to add IDDT to the agency's offerings. He believed that half of the agency's clients had co-occurring substance use disorders that adversely affected their recovery. He decided unilaterally that adding this service was essential. He contacted a well-known national consultant who provided IDDT training and scheduled a series of training sessions for all staff.

The consultant followed up by providing weekly and then monthly trainings, over the course of one year, covering all the basic steps of IDDT. Many of the clinicians were quite interested in the trainings. Some read materials provided by the consultant, and several tried to assess and treat substance abuse in their clients. When their clients' behaviors did not change quickly, however, the clinicians gradually gave up the efforts and returned to treatment practices they felt more skilled and successful in using. Their supervisors, managers, and quality improvement officers did not help them to continue IDDT. One year after the trainings, no trace of IDDT services could be found.

What happened to make this implementation fail? The CEO of the Lonesome Dove Agency made the decision to adopt IDDT without careful prior assessment. The CEO may have scanned medical records and learned that the rate of substance use disorders at his agency was 50 percent, or he may have just had a hunch, or he may have read a research report that claimed 50 percent was the typical rate in community mental health settings. Regardless, his belief led to the decision to implement IDDT throughout the agency, but he failed to consider the implications of his decision. He simply made an executive decision and announced that training in IDDT had been arranged. Let's see how he might have prepared differently.

Once the decision to adopt a new practice has been made, clinic leaders can take a number of concrete steps to prepare staff to implement it. The CEO and other clinical and administrative leaders should inform administrative, managerial, and supervisory staff about who will support the delivery of the new service and their role in the pending implementation. In turn, the clinical supervisors should discuss the pending implementation with the individuals who will provide the new service so that they can anticipate a change in the way they work and how it will affect them. Most of these activities fall within two domains, prioritization and leadership.

Prioritization

Prioritization means that the implementation is viewed as essential, and its success is understood to be the responsibility of all stakeholders. Fundamental to prioritizing the implementation of the new evidence-based practice is aligning participants' attitudes about the new practice. All stakeholders—from the state commissioner of mental health, to the CEO of the implementing agency, to the clinical supervisors, to the front-line clinicians, and to the clients and their families—must endorse the need for and acceptability of the new practice. In some cases, attitudes about the new practice will already be in line, but in other cases, key leaders will have to persuade others of the value of the practice. It is essential that leaders take responsibility early during the preparation stage to ensure buy-in among the clinical staff members who will implement the practice. Without clinical staff commitment well in advance of actual implementation, the chances of the implementation's success are greatly reduced. There will always be resistance to change, at both the clinical and organizational levels, and therefore, concerted effort must be expended to seek alignment of attitudes about the new practice. Some naysayers will not change their attitudes until they see proof that the new practice improves client outcomes or that it is financially viable. Some naysayers may never hold a positive attitude about the new practice, and it is up to leadership to ensure that these individuals are not in a position to sabotage the implementation.

> Prioritization means that the implementation's success is understood to be the responsibility of all stakeholders.

> The work of "selling" the new practice is never done.

The work of "selling" the new practice is never done. It must be continued through the implementation and maintenance stages as well. It should be easier once the practice is up and running, but the need to foster positive attitudes about the practice will not go away.

Another aspect of prioritization is the development of an understanding of the evidence-based practice to be implemented. This is not the same as training the clinical staff. Rather, it involves providing information about the new practice so that all stakeholders understand its fundamental principles and its promise to improve outcomes. For example, it is essential that clinical supervisors understand the practice before implementation begins. They will be responsible for preparing the frontline clinicians for the pending changes and for ensuring adherence to the principles of the evidence-based practice as it is being implemented. This understanding does not necessarily involve the specific details of the practice, but it must be sufficient to explain the nature of the practice and the need that it will serve. This is also the time to understand the nature of the organizational changes that are necessary for successful implementation. Only in this way can meaningful planning proceed. For example, it is necessary for agency leadership to understand the practice well enough to anticipate personnel requirements or changes to the agency's intake procedures.

Very little gets done in behavioral health care without a mechanism to pay for it. Implementation of even the best practices will not succeed without attention to funding. If the new service is reimbursable under current regulations, the way is paved. If there are not clear ways to pay for the service, expect a rocky road ahead. It is the job of leaders to have a clear sense of how to fund the new practice, not just in the short run, but in the long run as well.

These activities, part of what we call the domain of prioritization, are presented in table 1.

It is apparent that the CEO at Lonesome Dove did not attend to the tasks we identify as part of prioritization and jumped straight into training in IDDT. He mandated IDDT, but he did not foresee the need to recruit support for the upcoming changes. He did not allow time for an understanding of IDDT to develop among key clinical leaders, thereby enabling them to gain the support of the frontline clinicians. He did not look to the mental health authority for support, either for financial or policy backing. He did not look among his clinical staff for those who had experience with IDDT or other ways of treating substance abuse.

TABLE 1

The Domain of Prioritization

Implementation Dimension	Definition
Attitude	Clinic leaders offer expressions of support for the implementation of the evidence-based practice
Understanding	Understanding of the evidence-based practice is present or being sought
Mandate	The mental health authority requires that this evidence-based practice be offered
Money	Financial backing for the implementation of this evidence-based practice is available

In essence, he did not seek consensus about IDDT prior to making the decision to adopt it.

Neither did he ensure that staff members critical to the success of the implementation, especially the clinical supervisors, had an understanding of IDDT. Implementing a practice as challenging as IDDT requires additional work and responsibility for supervisors. Without their support, it is likely that the implementation will fail. Finally, he apparently did not evaluate the financial impact of implementing IDDT. Will substance abuse treatment in the mental health setting be reimbursed or is reimbursement for these services controlled by a separate addiction services division? The CEO had funding to provide training by an outside consultant, but that does not mean that he anticipated the many costs of implementing IDDT. IDDT requires regular assessments of substance abuse, the provision of individual- and group-based interventions, the development of advanced skills such as motivational interviewing and cognitive-behavioral treatment among all frontline clinicians, and time devoted to clinical supervision. Without considering how to pay for these activities, the CEO's decision to implement IDDT was not linked with the reality of implementing it.

Leadership

During the planning and prioritization of a new practice, several responsibilities fall to agency leaders. Other activities fall to them as well, specifically during preparation. These tasks and activities appear in table 2. At this stage, an EBP program leader should be designated and empowered to make decisions related to all aspects of implementation. The EBP program leader is the person responsible for the implementation of the practice. Ideally, this is the person who supervises the clinical staff who will implement the practice. Along the same lines, it is often helpful to identify those individuals who understand the value of the new practice and are willing to persuade others. These people are called

TABLE 2

The Domain of Leadership

Implementation Dimension	Definition
Responsibility	A program leader has the responsibility and authority to implement this evidence-based practice
Leadership Skills	Leadership skills for implementation and delivery of the evidence-based practice are present
Plan Enactment	A plan is in place for the implementation of the evidence-based practice
Engagement	Efforts are being made to build active support among other stakeholders for offering this evidence-based practice
Plan Sustaining	There is a plan for the sustained offering of this evidence-based practice
Change Culture	The agency culture is open to the changes needed to implement this evidence-based practice

"champions," and they take it upon themselves to advocate for the practice prior to and during its implementation. In some cases the EBP program leader will be the champion, but in other cases, the person may be an administrative leader or a frontline clinician. Many implementations have succeeded because of the energy and commitment of a local champion. Administrative leaders should identify and support champions who have the ability to influence others, as one strategy to create consensus for the value of implementing the new practice.

In addition, agency leaders are central to planning the implementation. In many cases, a leadership committee is formed to plan and oversee the implementation. This committee may contain agency leaders and the EBP program leader, but it may also contain clinical staff members and clients. In some cases, family members and community representatives are members of the leadership committee. This committee is where most of the decision making takes place during the preparation stage. The committee determines the scope of the implementation: How many practitioners will be trained to provide the new service, and how many of the eligible clients will be offered the service at the outset? This committee may look ahead to determine the staffing requirements for the new practice and the changes needed in the day-to-day workflow in order to accommodate the new practice. The committee may plan events to inform stakeholders within and outside the agency about the upcoming implementation. Furthermore, this committee should anticipate the types and amount of change that will be necessary at the organizational level in order to accommodate the new practice. In essence, the leadership committee both plans for the enactment of the new practice and anticipates possible barriers to successful implementation.

Agency leaders are central to planning the implementation.

There are two additional and related roles for leadership during the preparation phase. One is engaging key stakeholders in the planning process in order to ensure as much buy-in as possible. The more the key players demonstrate a positive attitude toward the evidence-based practice, understand its fundamentals and its promise to improve client outcomes, and engage in making the changes needed to implement it, the more smoothly the implementation will proceed.

The second role of leadership is to ensure that the culture of the organization is such that innovation and change are commonplace and anticipated with enthusiasm. The more that an agency prides itself on being agile and endorses a dynamic view of its services, the more easily a new practice can be implemented. This type of organizational culture does not happen suddenly or by mandate. It is a function of leadership style and an overt attempt by leaders to support innovation and change for the purpose of improving quality of care. But the culture of an organization is determined by more than the administrative leadership. It also depends on the attitudes and personality of clinical leaders and middle managers at all levels of the organization, and it depends intimately on the practitioners who will actually offer the new practice. This is not to say that a culture of change and innovation is necessary for successful implementation of an evidence-based practice, but the more that change and innovation are expected and facilitated, the more likely high-fidelity implementation will be achieved.

The CEO of the Lonesome Dove Agency not only failed to ensure that the implementation of IDDT was prioritized, but he also failed to provide the leadership associated with successful implementation. He did not attempt to engage relevant stakeholders in the process. He did not designate someone to lead the implementation and to be responsible for its success. Without some ownership of the decision to implement the practice or without anyone being empowered to plan for the implementation, why should the clinical leaders feel responsible for it? The CEO also did not form a leadership committee, which again means that responsibility for implementation was left unspecified, and another means to engage relevant stakeholders was not used.

In essence, the CEO exercised his right as leader of the agency to mandate the implementation of IDDT, but he did not enable the planning processes necessary for the implementation's success. Based on this case example, it appears that the CEO had not created a culture of change at the Lonesome Dove Agency. The choice to implement IDDT was made by an executive decision, and training came through an outside consultant. Both indicate that this agency does not have a culture that supports innovation. If the agency had such a culture, sufficient time would have been set aside to prioritize the implementation and properly plan for it at both the clinical and organizational levels. Although this case example seems extreme in its failure to prepare, it is not uncommon. At its heart is a failure to understand the scope of what's required to implement an evidence-based practice. Sweeping changes are not likely to occur based on a unilateral mandate and a rush to training. Without time to develop consensus around the decision to implement the evidence-based practice, without time for planning the implementation or assigning the responsibility for its success, it is unlikely that the practice will reach high fidelity and be maintained.

Implementation Stage

Once preparations have been made, it is time to launch the new initiative and to begin implementation. This stage may be viewed in two phases: starting up and striving for fidelity.

The implementation stage may be viewed in two phases: starting up and striving for fidelity.

Start-up often is marked by a significant event to kick off the implementation stage. Key stakeholders are invited to this public acknowledgment of the changes that are about to take place. Leaders extol the virtues of the new practice and lay out plans for the work ahead. Outside experts in the evidence-based practice, state-level consultant/trainers, and internal champions may speak about the practice. Introductory video presentations may also be offered as a means to inform everyone about the practice and to generate enthusiasm for the hard work ahead.

Most sites in the National Implementing Evidence-Based Practices Project held a kickoff event. Sites invited a wide range of stakeholders to a two- to three-hour event at which refreshments were served. There were speeches about the practice to be implemented and about the changes that were envisioned. Representatives from the mental health authority spoke in support of the evidence-based practice and described state-level support for it. The agency leadership, EBP program leaders, and an EBP champion were other speakers. PowerPoint presentations from the SAMHSA toolkits on the practices were used to reinforce the spoken content. Videos from the toolkits, which include client and clinician testimonials about the benefits of the practice, were also used to introduce the practice. Often the state-level trainer/consultant was introduced, and training schedules for clinical staff were announced. This kind of public event signifies the importance of the new practice and makes clear the priority placed on its successful implementation.

The other essential activity during start-up is staff training. Although the clinical staff will acquire most of their understanding through working with the practice, some sort of formal training for the EBP program leader, the clinical supervisor(s), and the frontline clinicians will be needed as well. How much training and in what form will vary by the evidence-based practice and by the composition of the clinical team. How much training to provide depends on the level of familiarity of the supervisors and practitioners with the practice, as well as their competence with the skills needed to implement it.

The form of the training can range from lectures by experts to online self-paced courses to one-on-one clinical supervision. Moreover, evidence-based practices like IDDT may require extensive training in the model and its constituent skills, because numerous practitioners are involved in providing a range of services. Alternatively, an evidence-based practice like IPS (also called supported employment) requires specialized and intensive training for vocational specialists but very little training for case managers, who provide support but do not deliver the service. It is often better to spread the training out over several months and to use multiple methods of instruction, adding complexity and nuance as practitioners gain experience with the practice.

Although formal training is often necessary, the greatest learning and skill acquisition often come through one-on-one clinical supervision. By reviewing cases and discussing problems and questions that arise when delivering the new service, the supervisor can shape and reinforce core elements of the practice, while at the same time pruning away extraneous activities and idiosyncratic adaptations.

This points to the crucial role of the supervisors during implementation and highlights the need to support them throughout this stage. Administrative leadership should provide time and resources for supervisors to become proficient in the evidence-based practice and to work closely with their staff members. This training will require more time during start-up and high-fidelity implementation, but it will also be required as long as the practice is offered. A technical assistance center, experienced colleagues, or learning collaboratives can help provide this support.

Ideally, supervisors and agency leaders should have had contact with a technical assistance center during the preparation stage, but if not, they should strongly consider it during the implementation stage. The technical assistance center can provide EBP training to clinical staff, consultation to the EBP program leader, and in-person supervision for the clinical supervisors. Agencies can consult with, or obtain training from, the technical assistance centers periodically during the implementation stage and as needed during the maintenance stage. Ongoing support will be critical to successful implementation, given the reality of how long it takes to achieve a high-fidelity implementation.

Learning collaboratives serve as another effective way for program leaders and clinical supervisors to learn about implementing the evidence-based practice and supervising staff using it. In a learning collaborative, peers join other practitioners at sites where the practice has been implemented in order to share experiences and to compare results such as fidelity scores and client outcomes. For example, facilitators at the state level may organize learning collaboratives, but participants from the implementing sites determine the activity and focus of the collaborative. It is also possible to form a learning collaborative with a wider range of participants across geographical borders. In these, members of the collaborative are from agencies across multiple states, and the facilitator is a national practitioner. For example, an existing learning collaborative for individual placement and support, facilitated by the developers and researchers of IPS at Dartmouth, involves leaders from mental health and vocational services from over a dozen states.

In these centers or collaboratives, participants learn from each other about how to overcome implementation barriers and how to maintain a high-fidelity implementation of the evidence-based practice. By comparing model fidelity and client outcomes across states and sites, participants are able to see what level of employment outcomes can be attained. This prompts low-performing states/sites to seek advice in order to improve outcomes, and over time the performance improves across all states/sites. The advantages of learning collaboratives are only beginning to be realized in behavioral health, but they appear to be powerful forces for achieving quality assurance.

Let's return to our case example of the Lonesome Dove Agency. The agency learned of new sources of funding and support for implementing IDDT. The agency tried again to prepare for and implement the evidence-based practice.

A Second Try at Implementation

Two years after the Lonesome Dove Agency failed to implement IDDT, the state's mental health and addiction programs combined to fund a center of excellence on IDDT. The center's technical assistance expert contacted Lonesome Dove's executive director and offered to meet and discuss the past attempt. She explained that the state's new plan was now based on an evidence-based approach to implementation. The state would reward a successful implementation with extra funding, and that implementation would begin with a six-month preparatory phase. The CEO of Lonesome Dove agreed to try to implement IDDT again.

During the preparatory phase, the technical assistance expert helped the agency create a leadership committee, revise medical records, hire a dual-disorders program leader, and train all supervisors in IDDT. She also helped the new dual-disorders program leader to review several existing programs, such as housing, skills training, and family psychoeducation, in order to help make the programs consistent with IDDT principles. She also encouraged the agency to revise credentialing procedures to allow for hiring people in recovery to help link clients with Alcoholics Anonymous and other Twelve Step groups.

Despite these preparations, Lonesome Dove encountered problems during implementation. The new program leader was asked to oversee the IDDT program as well as all case management, housing, and vocational services.

continued on next page

> *continued*
>
> Among these, he felt least confident in IDDT and therefore came to focus on the other programs and failed to prioritize IDDT. In the months following the IDDT expert's visit, the credentialing committee decided that the agency could not hire people in recovery. The medical records committee did not add substance use outcomes to mandatory records, and the agency did not start substance abuse groups. For the next year, fidelity reviews by the IDDT center's technical assistance expert revealed very poor implementation.

This time around, the state was much more involved, and preparations were more thorough and informed. A leadership committee was formed to steer the IDDT implementation, medical records were revised in anticipation of changes in assessment and documentation, an EBP program leader was hired, and supervisors were trained in IDDT. Because IDDT requires alignment with housing, skills training, and family psychoeducation services, the state technical assistance expert helped the EBP program leader to review these services and to make necessary changes. These preparations contrast with the first attempt to implement IDDT, and they provided Lonesome Dove with a solid foundation on which to build the new practice. Given state-level incentives and support, the implementation of IDDT had a higher priority, and the agency leadership took several positive steps to get it rolling. But the second attempt to employ IDDT also fell short. What went wrong? To understand, we'll need to consider two other domains of activities in implementing an evidence-based practice: workforce and workflow.

Workforce

For an evidence-based practice to take hold, the staff who will implement the practice need to be evaluated, trained, and supported. We identify these activities as staffing, personnel action, skill mastery, training, and supervision—activities that take place in the workforce domain (see table 3). These activities are added to the activities begun during the implementation stage and which we have listed under prioritization and leadership domains.

Staffing is about getting the right people in the various roles prescribed by the evidence-based practice. New staff members may need to be hired, and existing staff members may need to be reconfigured in order to meet the experience and skill requirements of the new practice.

TABLE 3

The Domain of Workforce

Implementation Dimension	Definition
Staffing	Attempts are being made to meet the staffing requirements of the evidence-based practice
Personnel Action	Personnel problems that detract from implementation and delivery of the evidence-based practice are addressed
Skill Mastery	The skills needed by practitioners to offer the evidence-based practice are present or being sought
Training	Training in the evidence-based practice is being offered
Supervision	Clinical supervision of the evidence-based practice is being offered

Despite the difficulty in doing so, some staff members may have to be moved to other positions within the agency or terminated from the agency. We have seen too many implementations languish because leaders were reluctant to make the changes in personnel needed to achieve a high-fidelity implementation. It benefits no one, especially the consumers of services, if staff members with negative attitudes or weak skills are allowed to remain on the job.

It seems obvious that supervisors, including the EBP program leaders and clinical staff members, will need training in the evidence-based practice. What is not obvious is how to provide such training. Given the high rate of turnover among case managers and other frontline clinical staff, it may make sense to train the supervisors and then enable them to train their staff members. Although training of supervisors may take several forms, it may be best to provide a minimum of "classroom" training and the maximum possible of "field" training. That is, it may be most effective to have an outside expert provide ongoing training and supervision of the program leader and clinical supervisors, as the agency implements the practice with the initial group of clients. The clinical supervisors, in turn, would provide introductory training to the clinical staff members and then supervise them closely during the first six to twelve months of implementation. Avoiding mind-numbing hours of classroom instruction and focusing instead on the acquisition and

> Workforce: it may be best to provide a minimum of "classroom" training and the maximum possible of "field" training.

enactment over time of specific principles will ensure that the evidence-based practice is more effectively learned.

This model of close supervision over time is also the way to ensure mastery of the skills needed to implement the evidence-based practice. For example, IDDT requires motivational interviewing and cognitive-behavioral treatment for successful implementation. In order to deliver IDDT, frontline clinicians should have acquired these skills and know when to use them. Therefore, high-fidelity implementation of IDDT requires learning about its principles, structural features, and core services, but it also requires mastery of the clinical skills that are required to offer the core services. (As discussed in chapter 4, one can argue that one set of skills comprises the core of various evidence-based practices.)

As seen in our case example, the second attempt to implement IDDT at the Lonesome Dove Agency got off to a good start but did not succeed. Was the failure due in part to lack of attention to staff support and training, what we call the workforce domain? Although the agency hired an IDDT program leader and the state's technical assistance program provided support, his role was not singularly devoted to the implementation of IDDT. The dilution of his responsibilities precluded his learning the principles of IDDT and the core skills that accompany the practice. Consequently, he fell back on those programs with which he felt most comfortable to the detriment of IDDT. Although not said in the case report, the program leader no doubt failed to provide adequate supervision to the clinical supervisors and staff members. Without this support, staff would be left with an inadequate understanding of IDDT and a lack of mastery of the core skills that IDDT requires. This training would have also helped the credentialing committee. Its refusal to hire people in recovery from substance abuse resulted in a core component of IDDT (i.e., peer support) not being implemented.

Workflow

Whereas implementing agencies will readily decide to bring in experts to train the clinical staff in the evidence-based practice, they may not consider the need for consultation on the organizational changes that will be needed to succeed. It is important to remember that implementation of an evidence-based practice requires changes at two levels: at the service delivery/clinical level and at the management/administrative level. An agency's workflow needs to be reviewed and revised. Workflow refers to the physical setting and administrative details that are part of any practice in behavioral health, such as the role of support staff, structure of meetings, documentation required, and policies (see table 4). Thoughtful attention to each of these elements of activity will facilitate implementation. The goal is to make the flow of work such that doing the right thing—that is, the evidence-based practice—becomes the path of least resistance. It should be harder to work in the old ways and easier to follow the principles of the new practice. Consultants in organizational change can help agencies redesign their workflow to achieve this goal.

TABLE 4
The Domain of Workflow

Implementation Dimension	Definition
Staff Meetings	A meeting structure that supports the evidence-based practice is present
Documentation	Documentation practices support the evidence-based practice
Support Staff	Support staff function to support the evidence-based practice
Physical Environment	The physical environment supports the implementation of the evidence-based practice
Policies	Policies supporting the evidence-based practice are present

Meetings can be restructured to focus on the implementation and scheduled so as not to interfere with the delivery of the evidence-based practice. Documentation can be simplified and aligned with the new practice. For example, billing systems can require justification for *not* delivering an evidence-based practice when it is warranted. Electronic clinical support systems can guide clinicians to evidence-based practices, rather than old ways of delivering services, and enable record keeping that supports the new practices.

Frontline clinicians need time to deliver effective services rather than being required to fill out endless forms. Electronic medical record systems, in which billing and clinical support systems may be embedded, can facilitate the use of evidence-based practices, although gains in efficiency are not guaranteed unless these systems are also streamlined and made less burdensome for the practitioners. It is essential that information related to EBP fidelity and client outcomes is collected routinely and becomes an integral part of supervision. Collection of these data and their feedback to practitioners can become part of routine practice and fit within the workflow.

If the evidence-based practice is team-based, office space can be reconfigured to put clinicians on teams in proximity with one another. If staff members assume new roles due to the implementation of an evidence-based practice, their offices may also have to be reassigned in order to facilitate working with others. A new job in an old office may not work well. In addition, administrative staff should be trained to support the new practice. They can help with recruitment of clients, scheduling, preparation of clients for office visits, and documentation. Finally, agency policies can be modified to enable the new practice and to keep it as a high priority. Policies that hinder access to the evidence-based practice or that cause problems for full implementation should be questioned. New policies may be needed in order to provide solutions to problems that arise due to implementing a new practice.

It appears that some criteria for establishing a good workflow were overlooked in the IDDT implementation at the Lonesome Dove Agency. The agency may have had a standing policy against credentialing people in recovery, but by not addressing this policy, the agency failed to add an important component of IDDT: peer counselors. The agency's failure to hire people in recovery was not only a failure to address workforce issues but also a failure to align the agency's policy with the practice of IDDT.

The agency's documentation procedures also caused problems. The medical records committee did not add substance abuse outcomes to routine documentation. Thus, clinical supervisors had no way to evaluate progress in this key client outcome. This omission seriously impeded effective supervision.

Perhaps most significantly, the agency failed to engage someone from the state's technical assistance center as a consultant on organizational change. The case report notes that the center of excellence had an evidence-based approach to implementation, but it's not clear that this approach was used at Lonesome Dove. If the technical support to an agency is solely devoted to training and support for the clinical changes without any attention to the accompanying organizational and administrative changes, the implementation is crippled from the outset.

Training and consultation in both arenas go hand in hand, and special assistance may be needed in both of them. The elements of an organization and its administrative functions that support implementation of new practices are described in the workforce and workflow domains.

Testing Fidelity to the EBP Model

Throughout the implementation stage, agency practitioners should keep an eye on the fidelity to the EBP model. The practice's faithfulness to the model will be the primary means by which the success of the initial implementation is judged. In order for a practice to be designated as evidence-based, it has been rigorously tested in randomized controlled trials in a variety of settings and with a range of clients, and in all these settings it has been shown to achieve desired client outcomes. The logic then is that if a site implements the evidence-based practice with high fidelity, it will achieve the same desired outcomes. The familiar refrain that "our clients are different so we need to adapt the evidence-based practice" is seldom valid and should be avoided at the outset of implementation. The tendency to want to adapt an evidence-based practice is common, as clinicians think that they know what works best for their clients. Nevertheless, the guiding principle should be to implement the practice according to the model and then, once the practice has stabilized as a high-fidelity implementation, to look at client outcomes to determine how to improve the practice further.

An EBP fidelity scale reveals how well an implementation falls in line with accepted practice, and it can provide a road map for the implementation stage. The scale measures all the key components of the practice, and it provides specific targets for each component. Conducting a fidelity assessment at the outset and at regular intervals provides specific guidance on implementing a particular evidence-based practice. It is recommended that fidelity assessments be conducted by outside evaluators, who can look at an implementation impartially and in comparison to other implementations that they have assessed. States often have trained raters for this purpose.

In a typical fidelity assessment, raters visit the site for a day. They review documentation, interview supervisors and frontline clinicians, talk to clients, observe service delivery, and so forth. The raters meet afterward to reconcile their ratings and to prepare a fidelity report. The report should indicate how the site is doing on each item on the fidelity assessment. The EBP program leader and the leadership committee (or whoever is overseeing the implementation) can use the fidelity report to plan implementation activities for the coming months. Those in charge of the implementation can use the report to note areas of high fidelity and to encourage supervisors and clinicians to keep doing what they are doing in these areas. Barriers to achieving a high-fidelity implementation are also identified, and strategies to overcome them are proposed. Maintaining a focus on fidelity to the EBP model makes the path to successful implementation clear. Paying attention to fidelity during the implementation stage reduces the temptation to adapt the practice to fit local conditions.

A focus on fidelity to the EBP model makes the path to successful implementation clear.

The Lonesome Dove Agency, despite its renewed efforts, did not attend to fidelity. The agency did not employ people in recovery and did not start substance abuse groups, another failure in fidelity. Regardless of the reasons for these decisions, they indicate a lack of attention to the key principles of IDDT. Without full implementation of an evidence-based practice, the expectation is that the practice will not achieve its promise of improved client outcomes. Implementing a new practice is hard, and if the hard work does not show gains for clinicians and clients, the new practice will probably fail, as enthusiasm and adherence wane. Such was the case at Lonesome Dove, as fidelity assessments throughout the first year indicated poor implementation.

A Third Try

After a year of watching his agency floundering, Lonesome Dove's executive director decided to renew efforts to implement IDDT. Following the guidance from technical assistance more closely this time, he added an IDDT program director with directly relevant experience and whose only responsibility was to oversee IDDT. He insisted that the medical records committee include substance use outcomes, that the credentialing committee work out a compromise to allow hiring people in recovery as links to the local Alcoholics Anonymous and Twelve Step groups in the community, and that the clinical director provide incentives to clinicians to start IDDT groups. Training began anew.

All clinicians received two days of didactic training combined with practice in live interactions. Subsequently, each staff member identified five clients with co-occurring substance use disorders, discussed these cases with their supervisors, and met with the clients and supervisor together for field-based supervision. This process continued for six months before clinicians were

continued on next page

> *continued*
>
> expected to screen all their clients for substance abuse or dependence and to monitor their assessments and progress using standardized forms. Supervisors and team leaders monitored outcomes as well as gave continuing regular supervision. One year later, the state's technical assistance expert scored Lonesome Dove in the high-fidelity range for IDDT. The program was implemented well and became a source of pride for the agency.

Maintenance Stage

Once assessments indicate that the practice has been implemented at the desired level of fidelity, the practice has moved from the implementation stage to the maintenance stage. In many ways this is the most difficult stage. Preparation involves planning the steps needed to begin offering the new practice and anticipating any challenges to its implementation. It is a time when enthusiasm is growing for the new practice, with its promise to improve client outcomes. The implementation stage is an exciting time, when lots of energy is devoted to making the necessary changes at the organizational and clinical levels. The clinical staff acquire new knowledge and skills, and attention is focused on the work that they are doing. Clients may be encouraged by the new practice and have renewed hope that their lives will be improved by the changes in their services. The maintenance stage is when the new practice becomes part of the routine. Its novelty has worn off for the practitioners, who are now expected to maintain its quality and value to clients. Its prominence among the many services offered begins to fade, and practitioners begin to look down the road to see what the next change in practice will be.

One way to ensure continued enthusiasm for and quality of the evidence-based practice is to commit to reinforcing the new practice. In our work, we see the importance of reinforcing practices, and therefore, we have added the domain of reinforcement to the activities of prioritization, leadership, workforce, and workflow that are in place and that have brought the practice to the point of maintenance (see table 5).

Fidelity assessments play an important role during the implementation stage, but the need for fidelity assessment continues as long as the evidence-based practice is offered. There are always ways to improve the implementation of a practice, and it is useful to be reminded of those areas where no progress has been made or where adherence to the core elements of the practice has eroded. Maintaining a high-fidelity

TABLE 5
The Domain of Reinforcement

Implementation Dimension	Definition
Penetration	Measures of program penetration are collected and used to improve the evidence-based practice.
Outcome Monitoring	Client outcomes are collected and monitored in order to improve the evidence-based practice.
Fidelity	Measures of fidelity are collected and used to improve the evidence-based practice.
Rewards	Success is celebrated in order to reinforce the evidence-based practice.
Credentialing	Programs are credentialed to reinforce the evidence-based practice.
Feedback	Feedback from practitioners and clients is solicited and used to monitor and improve the evidence-based practice.

evidence-based practice is one sure way to increase the likelihood of gains for clients. When maintaining a practice, we recommend that fidelity assessments be conducted by outside raters on a periodic basis. However, the agency may decide that its quality assurance staff will conduct interim assessments. Staff may use the fidelity scale in these assessments, but, in addition, checklists such as those presented in chapter 3 may be effective tools for ensuring that the processes within the evidence-based practice are maintained.

In addition to fidelity assessments, a concerted effort should be made to collect client outcomes. Whereas fidelity concerns the processes of implementation, outcome monitoring concerns the effectiveness of the practice. Quality cannot be improved or maintained without the concrete feedback that outcome monitoring provides. Ideally, this client outcome data would have been gathered beginning at the implementation stage, but gathering this information is often put off while other changes are being made. Nevertheless, once the agency has begun to maintain the practice, for continued improvement and for effective clinical supervision, it is critical to collect carefully targeted outcomes on a periodic basis.

> Quality cannot be improved or maintained without the concrete feedback that outcome monitoring provides.

If you are implementing supported employment, you can track work outcomes for your clients. If you are implementing IDDT, you can track substance use outcomes and participants' stages of recovery from substance abuse. The principle is really quite simple: you can't change an outcome that you don't observe.

The key guideline is to keep the outcome assessment simple, at least at the beginning. Pick a few outcomes of interest to clinicians and clients and focus on measuring them well.

Collecting client outcomes is only the start, for it is the monitoring of outcomes that really matters. Monitoring outcomes can take many forms, but the most useful form for maintaining an evidence-based practice is having supervisors bring outcome summaries to their meetings with their staff members. Supervisors can report client outcomes at the individual and group levels over time. This reporting provides a means to guide practice. The performance of teams and individuals can be compared. This enables reinforcement for high performers and remediation for low performers. Insightful discussions can arise when actual outcomes are viewed and discussed. Targets can be set for desired rates of client outcomes, and the tracking of those outcomes over time enables evaluation of the success of the practice and modifications to it. For example, supervisors of vocational specialists who are delivering supported employment can use employment outcomes (days worked, time to first job, longest time worked, etc.) to monitor the performance of the specialists. Those who are getting good outcomes can suggest strategies for the low performers to try, thereby encouraging a high standard for outcomes among all vocational specialists. For programs implementing IDDT, days of use of alcohol and drugs can be monitored over time for each client and summarized periodically for review by supervisors and frontline clinicians. The basic idea is one of the fundamentals of behaviorism: you can only change that which you monitor. The simple act of tracking client outcomes over time will improve practice, and these gains will reinforce the use of the evidence-based practice.

Moreover, monitoring client outcomes provides meaningful insights on how to achieve greater gains. If the implementation of a practice has stabilized at high fidelity, monitoring outcomes can be a way to test adaptations of the model that may result in better outcomes. Our belief is that initial implementation of an evidence-based practice should focus on fidelity as the measure of success, because reaching high fidelity is the best way to ensure good outcomes for clients. But after a practice has reached high-fidelity implementation, it makes sense to add a focus on client outcomes as a means to guide modifications of the practice in order to achieve the highest level of outcomes possible. Feedback from frontline clinicians and from clients may suggest practice improvements that might enhance outcomes. With the analysis that can be provided by outcome data, managers and supervisors have a powerful argument in favor of using those practice adaptations that have been shown to lead to improvements in outcomes, as well as evidence against using those adaptations that do not improve outcomes. The guiding principle is to be systematic and thoughtful when making adaptations so that the results from outcome monitoring can be used strategically to add changes to or prune elements of the EBP model. We emphasize that adaptations to an evidence-based practice are not advised during initial implementation. They should only be considered once a high-fidelity implementation has been attained and when there is room for improvement in client outcomes.

Another means of sustaining an evidence-based practice is encouraging its wide dissemination, or what is called its penetration. The term "penetration" refers to the proportion of eligible clients who are actually able to access the practice. It is common for the initial implementation to involve only a few clinicians or one or two teams of clinicians. The initial limited implementation of a practice helps to contain the upheaval caused by a new practice and to enable its delivery to go well. Once the practice has reached high fidelity and is being maintained, leaders and practitioners can turn their attention to expanding the practice. It's a good rule to start small and establish a high-fidelity implementation, but the long-term goal should be to offer the practice to all eligible clients. This means that while some clinicians are maintaining the practice, other clinicians may be beginning to implement it. Strong and engaged leadership, at multiple levels, will be required to coordinate the activities needed to expand the evidence-based practice. The experience of the initial adopters can be used to facilitate the practice's growth, while fidelity and outcome monitoring can gauge progress being made with the expanded use of the practice.

Research has shown time and time again that positive reinforcement is the best way to change and to maintain a behavior. When seeking to maintain an evidence-based practice, leaders should not pass up any opportunity to praise those who are doing exceptional work, especially during the maintenance stage, when the luster of the new practice has

> Another means of sustaining an evidence-based practice is encouraging its wide dissemination.

worn off. Everyone likes a pat on the back. It makes people feel valued, and it helps to maintain enthusiasm for the job and quality of the work. Public acknowledgment and awards to recognize quality are ways leaders can show appreciation for the efforts of their staff members.

Leaders can also acknowledge staff members' achievements by encouraging them to seek credentials for competence in an evidence-based practice. This type of certification spotlights achievement and competence of the workforce, and it reinforces professionalism. The more that clinical staff members are praised, rewarded, and credentialed, the more confident they will be in delivering the new practice. And the more that the practice becomes second nature, the easier it will be to maintain. In addition, once a nucleus of experienced and skilled clinicians has developed, it will be easier to train and supervise new staff members, thereby further enabling maintenance of the practice.

Keeping the successful implementation of the practice a high priority will be a constant job. As mentioned earlier, during maintenance of the practice, the activities within all five implementation domains will be under way. In order to keep staff morale high and to ensure continued funding of the evidence-based practice, leaders and champions will have to continue to advocate for the practice. Workflow and workforce issues will also need continued attention. Today's community behavioral health workforce turns over at an alarming rate—somewhere near 50 percent of providers leave the workforce every two years. This means that the need for training and supervision will be constant throughout the life of any evidence-based practice. Planners should take this into account when forecasting the demands of a new practice. Workflow should undergo periodic evaluation to ensure that the multiple services offered by an agency do not collide with or hinder each other. Attention to the practical and administrative details of coexisting services will streamline workflow and provide time for actual delivery of services.

As should be obvious by now, the responsibilities and activities of leaders are crucial and ongoing during all stages of implementation of an evidence-based practice. Leaders can be key to a successful implementation, but they can also, unfortunately, become a serious obstacle. With a change in leadership, agencies can drift from established high-fidelity practices. In one instance at Lonesome Dove, a new executive director canceled technical assistance and fidelity visits from the state implementation expert and did not rehire people in recovery. The final blow came when the dual-disorders program director left the agency and was replaced by someone who did not have expertise in IDDT. The leadership failed to reinforce the practice. Over the next year, the lack of support led to a decline in IDDT supervision and an increase in staff turnover. The commitment to IDDT soon faded away.

While not enough can be said about the importance of leadership to program success, it seems that little has been determined about how one should lead. A mountain of books and reams of data address leadership styles, but concrete, practical advice on how to be an effective leader is scarce. There is no simple answer to the question of what makes an effective leader. It turns out that leaders with different styles can achieve comparable results. Effectiveness has more to do with what leaders do than with the style in which they do it. For example, it matters less whether a leader has an authoritarian or consensus-building style than whether that leader provides a vision, empowers others, and rewards success. One bit of advice would be for leaders to learn from others and never to be content with the belief that they know how to lead.

Learning collaboratives are one way that leaders join together around the single purpose of improving performance. Whether formal or informal, learning collaboratives let agency leaders share information, both experiential and empirical, with their peers and learn from each other about effective versus ineffective ways to implement and maintain an evidence-based practice.

The Lonesome Dove Agency's third attempt to implement and maintain IDDT was much more successful. This time much more attention was paid to the activities that ensure successful implementation. An experienced IDDT program leader was hired, substance use outcomes were tracked in medical records, and policies were changed to enable people in recovery to be hired. An experiential model of training was used to ensure that practitioners were knowledgeable and skilled before their caseload of IDDT clients was expanded. Practitioners screened all of their clients for possible substance abuse or dependence, in order to determine who should be offered IDDT. Client outcomes were collected and used during supervision, and an outside expert rated the IDDT program at high fidelity after one year.

Even though the CEO of the Lonesome Dove Agency made mistakes, he did not lose his commitment to IDDT. He persevered, learned from his mistakes, and eventually succeeded in implementing an effective IDDT program. But the existence of a high-fidelity program in no way ensures its maintenance when faced with changes in leadership or other critical factors, such as changes in financing and state-level policies. Unfortunately, those who lose the most in these circumstances are those clients who need IDDT in order to support their recovery from substance abuse.

Summary

In the Lonesome Dove Agency's first try at implementing IDDT, the agency failed at preparation. The CEO learned from this failure to prepare, but the agency fell short at following through on the tasks of implementation. In the third effort, the agency attained a high-fidelity implementation of IDDT, but as we've noted, if the agency and its leadership wish to remain successful, they will need to make concerted efforts to maintain the practice.

These case examples illustrate the stages of implementation. While they show how easily things can go wrong, we hope they also suggest the steps that can be taken to avoid or correct problems. The examples are drawn from our experience, and the mistakes are common. The advice we've presented here applies as well to implementations of any of the five evidence-based practices that we studied in the National Implementing Evidence-Based Practices Project. These issues are not unique to IDDT. In hindsight, it may seem easy to identify ways to better implement a new practice. The challenge is to anticipate problems and avoid mistakes.

In this chapter, we've illustrated how implementation of an evidence-based practice moves through three stages: preparation, implementation, and maintenance. Each stage can be defined by the tasks required and the activities of leaders and clinical staff members. Five domains described in this chapter encompass the activities that occur across the three stages of implementation. Prioritization of the practice and leadership are critical during all three stages. Workforce and workflow activities begin in the implementation stage and continue through the maintenance stage. Reinforcement activities help to maintain a practice.

These stages and domains, or the tasks and activities within them, provide a way to think comprehensively and in advance about the task of implementation. But, in implementing an evidence-based practice, few specific and necessary activities can be identified. The framework we have provided can serve only as a guideline. There is no simple, proven formula for successful implementation of an evidence-based practice. Each implementation is different, because the context and people involved are different.

For additional help with implementing a practice and carrying out the changes needed at the clinical and organizational levels, we suggest that implementers seek advice and support from technical assistance centers or other similar resources such as implementation toolkits. (For examples and further information, see Recommended Reading and Resources.) These resources will help ensure that your agency can set realistic expectations about what you can achieve and the necessary activities for implementing an evidence-based practice.

Evidence-based practices have been shown to be effective and to advance areas of treatment or rehabilitation that best support recovery. The rewards to be found in successfully implementing an evidence-based practice are many, but none more so than the improvements these practices can encourage in the lives of your clients. As challenging as achieving a high-fidelity implementation may be, you can take satisfaction in knowing that the practices are making a real difference in the lives of the people you serve.

2

Implementation Measures

AN ESSENTIAL INGREDIENT to successful implementation of an evidence-based practice is systematically tracking key process indicators and making improvements based on these indicators. Put simply, quality improvement entails measurement, feedback, and corrective action. The critical role of measurement in implementation is apparent in instances when an agency "flies blind" without any rigorous attempt to gauge its implementation process or extent of successful implementation. But what should program leaders measure? When well-established practical measures already exist, then leaders should use these.

A Framework for Measuring Implementation of Evidenced-Based Practices

When evaluating an implementation, we consider the organization's readiness to use the practice, the practice's fidelity to the model, the availability and dissemination of the practice (or its penetration), and client outcomes. We recommend collecting data in all these areas. By *organizational readiness,* we mean the capacity of the organization to implement the practice. Is there sufficient staffing or the capacity to hire appropriate staff? Are there predictable funding sources to pay for the services and the means to train and supervise staff in the practice? Another way to think about organizational readiness is to consider whether the organization will be able to overcome common barriers to implementation. We recommend using checklists to measure organizational readiness. Readiness checklists serve as road maps. Completion of most or all of the items on the checklist signals that an agency is more likely to be adequately prepared, while significant gaps in the checklist (especially for critical elements) signal the need for more preparatory work. It is most helpful if completing a checklist prompts program leaders to develop an action plan, which they then monitor and revise over time.

Agencies should also assess the success of the practice and its implementation. They should look to client outcomes and how faithfully their program emulates the EBP model. They should consider how widely used the practice is among clients; that is, the number of eligible clients participating in the evidence-based practice suggests the *penetration* of the practice. We measure penetration by the proportion of clients receiving the practice. It is the number of clients participating divided by the number who are eligible and would benefit from the program.

By *fidelity,* we mean the degree to which the program, as implemented, adheres to the guidelines and principles defining the evidence-based practice. The term *client outcomes* refers to the outcomes specific to the practice, based on effectiveness research.

In this chapter, we provide a framework indicating the major types of indicators we recommend measuring. We also provide a list of implementation measures that agency leaders, state planners, and researchers might consult when implementing an evidence-based practice. Some of these measures function as standardized, normed instruments that can be used without modification, depending on the practice under consideration. Other measures are included because they provide examples of what might be measured and how it might be measured.

Of the instruments intended for direct application, many are appropriate for quality improvement purposes. Some help identify barriers to adoption or organizational readiness, while others help evaluators monitor the degree to which practices have been successfully implemented.

In selecting measures, we generally recommend using measures that are specific to the evidence-based practice, rather than general-purpose implementation scales. EBP-specific measures are more sensitive to the practice being implemented than are general-purpose measures. However, the downside to this recommendation is that many EBP-specific measures have not yet been created, which means that program leaders may need to develop their own scales. For advice in developing a new fidelity scale, we recommend consulting a toolkit on fidelity scale development that has a step-by-step guide to this process (Bond et al. 2000).

Commonly Used Implementation Measures

As shown in table 6, implementation measures can be divided into two categories: those that evaluate factors that influence implementation and those that measure implementation outcomes. The first category refers to predictors of successful implementation and maintenance while the second category refers to indicators of a successful implementation. We also distinguish between two broad types of interventions or practices: program-level practices (also referred to as team-based interventions) and practitioner-led practices. The team-based interventions involve a group of practitioners who together deliver the EBP services, and practitioner interventions are delivered by an individual practitioner, typically in the form of individual psychotherapy or counseling.

In this chapter, we give examples of measures for program-level and practitioner-level evidence-based practices. We also identify several organizational and system-level measures. Finally, we note several important aspects of the implementation process for which there are no existing measures that we can recommend for use. When no appropriate measures exist, we recommend that program implementers develop simple and direct indicators specific to their practice. Table 6, included in this chapter and on the CD-ROM, provides an overview of the implementation measures discussed (see pages 32–33).

Measuring Factors Influencing Implementation

In this section, we examine a variety of factors influencing the implementation process. We begin with two broad frameworks measuring barriers, facilitators, and strategies influencing implementation. Next, we describe practitioner attitudes toward adoption of the practice, the practice's acceptability to clients, organizational readiness, and the role of leadership at the governmental/funder level.

Implementation Factor Frameworks

A way to identify factors influencing the success of an implementation is to evaluate a broad range of organizational factors. As part of the National Implementing Evidence-Based Practices Project, we developed the National EBP Project Implementation Framework, which consists of a comprehensive set of categories used to classify implementation factors. Factors identified include the barriers to implementation and strategies and facilitators promoting implementation. As described in chapter 1,

TABLE 6
Implementation Measures

Measures of Factors Influencing Implementation

Area of Inquiry	Instrument or Factor Measured	Unit of Measure	Data Sources	Mode of Measurement	Time Required	Reliability of Instrument	Validity	Citation*
Comprehensive Implementation Factor Frameworks	National EBP Project Implementation Framework	program	multiple stakeholders at site level	qualitative data collection	extensive	interrater	associated with EBP fidelity	(Torrey et al. 2012)
	Rogers–Rütten Conceptual Framework	program	program leaders	checklist	brief	internal consistency	one component correlated with EBP fidelity	(Bowen et al. 2010)
Acceptability to Clients	dropout rate	program	clients	agency records	minimal	variable	---	---
Organizational Readiness	AIMS Team-Building Tool	organization	intervention team	self-assessment	not reported	---	---	(AIMS Center 2011)
	Agency Readiness for IPS-SE Checklist	organization	practitioners, program leaders	site visit	one day	---	---	(Swanson and Becker 2011)
Governmental/ Funder Leadership	SHAY	state	state/government administrators	site visit	one day or more	interrater	associated with EBP fidelity	(Finnerty et al. 2009)

Implementation Outcomes

Area of Inquiry	Instrument or Factor Measured	Unit of Measure	Data Sources	Mode of Measurement	Time Required	Reliability of Instrument	Validity	Citation*
Adoption	Adoption Decision Factor Survey	organization	key informants	interview	not reported	---	---	(Panzano and Roth 2006)
Penetration	percentage enrolled/eligible	organization	agency	agency records	variable	---	---	(National EBP Project)
Maintenance	Dartmouth Sustainability Interview	program	program leaders	phone interview	40 minutes	---	---	(Bond, McHugo, Becker et al. 2012)
	Decision to De-Adopt Index	organization	agency decision makers	structured interview	62 items (variable time to complete interviews)	---	---	(Massatti et al. 2008)

Fidelity	GOI	program	program	site visit	half-day	interrater	associated with EBP fidelity	(Bond et al. 2009)
	DDCAT	organization	organization	site visit	one day	interrater, internal consistency	criterion-related (associated with client-level admission data)	(McGovern et al. 2007)
	DDCMHT	organization	organization	site visit	one day	interrater, internal consistency	convergent/discriminant (associated with IDDT Fidelity Scale)	(Gotham et al. 2010)
	DDCHCS	organization	organization	site visit	one day	interrater, internal consistency	---	---
	SE Fidelity Scale	program	program	site visit	1.5 days	interrater	discriminative and predictive	(Becker et al. 2011)
	DACTS	program	program	site visit	one day	interrater	discriminative	(Teague et al. 1998)
	TMACT	program	program	site visit	two days	interrater	discriminative	(Monroe-DeVita et al. 2011)
	IMR Fidelity Scale	program	program	site visit	one day	interrater	---	(Mueser et al. 2005)
	IT-IS	practitioner	practitioner	audiotape ratings	1 hour per session	interrater	discriminative	(McGuire et al. 2012)
	ITRS for MI Fidelity Monitoring	practitioner	practitioner	audiotape ratings	1 hour per session	interrater	---	(Martino et al. 2008)
	YACS	practitioner	practitioner	audiotape or observational ratings of therapy sessions	1 hour per session	interrater, internal consistency, test-retest	criterion-related (associated with therapeutic alliance, retention)	(Carroll et al. 2000)
	MedTEAM Organizational and Prescriber Fidelity Scales	organization and prescribers	organizational leader/medical director and organization documents; patient medical records (for prescriber)	interview; review of paper and/or electronic documents	1–2 hours for organization; 36 minutes per patient chart (paper charts)	interrater, test-retest	---	(SAMHSA 2010)

Note: Blank cells in the above matrix indicate that no information is currently available to the authors.

*Cited sources appear in references for chapter 2.

Acronyms: AIMS: Advancing Integrated Mental Health Solutions; SE: Supported Employment; SHAY: State Health Authority Yardstick; GOI: General Organizational Index; DDCAT: Dual Diagnosis Capability in Addiction Treatment; DDCMHT: Dual Diagnosis Capability in Mental Health Treatment; DDCHCS: Dual Diagnosis Capability in Health Care Settings; DACTS: Dartmouth Assertive Community Treatment Scale; TMACT: Tool for Measurement of Assertive Community Treatment; IMR: Illness Management and Recovery; IT–IS: IMR Treatment-Integrity Scale; ITRS: Independent Tape Rating Scale; MI: motivational interviewing; YACS: Yale Adherence and Competence Scale.

this framework consists of twenty-six categories of implementation activities grouped into five implementation domains (Torrey, Bond, McHugo, and Swain 2012). These implementation domains are prioritization, leadership, workforce, workflow, and reinforcement. This framework is very flexible and can be adapted for use with a wide range of practices. But the methods used in the National Implementing Evidence-Based Practices Project to collect information on implementation domains were labor intensive. A checklist version of this framework would be more suitable for typical implementation projects.

Another framework for identifying factors predictive of a successful implementation is the Rogers–Rütten Conceptual Framework. Developed as a synthesis of the work of two theorists (Bowen et al. 2010), this twenty-one-item checklist consists of six components or features to be evaluated. These components—listed under the headings Relative Advantage, Compatibility, Goals, Funding Obligation, Service Obligation, and Resources—describe the perception of the evidence-based practice by the staff at the agency implementing the practice. For example, one item measuring Relative Advantage asks, "To what extent do you agree with the following? This evidence-based practice takes a long time to implement compared to interventions that are not evidence-based practices." Program leaders rate the responses to these items. As reported in one study, the first component, Relative Advantage, was significantly correlated with EBP fidelity (Bowen et al. 2010).

Because of their critical importance, two implementation factors that warrant special mention are funding and leadership. To fully implement and maintain a practice, an agency must have sufficient funding. In fact, the availability of funding is widely recognized as a key factor influencing the success of an implementation. Funding should cover both the costs of start-up (e.g., initial training, new equipment, and materials needed for the practice) and the ongoing costs of providing services. It is also important that sources of funding are predictable and permanent. How services are funded—for example, whether they are fee-for-service, capitation, or pay-for-performance—also influences the viability of a practice. The number of funding sources needed and the requirements for receipt of funding are still other critical factors in implementing and maintaining an evidence-based practice. Unfortunately, there are no standardized measures to assess the adequacy of funding. Because evidence-based practices differ widely in per-client costs and in typical sources of funding, and because funding differs so widely across states, it is probably best to individualize assessment in this area.

Many studies have indicated that leadership shown by program leaders and agency administrators is instrumental to successful implementation (Torrey, Bond, McHugo, and Swain 2012). Leaders provide resources, problem-solve, and provide inspiration and encouragement. Unfortunately, none of the existing quantitative measures of leadership adequately captures the crucial roles leaders play in implementing evidence-based practices, and therefore we cannot recommend any specific scales in this area.

Practitioner Attitudes toward Adoption of Practice

One factor influencing the successful adoption and continued use of a practice is its acceptability to practitioner and program leaders. The acceptability of a practice reflects the assumptions, beliefs, and values of the people responsible for implementing a practice and their perceptions about the ease with which it can be adopted and used. It also presumably reflects the practice's compatibility with the practitioners' therapeutic orientation, attitudes, skills, and knowledge.

We do not recommend using any of the published measures of practitioner attitudes about evidence-based practices because they are not specific enough. There's currently not enough evidence on the predictive value or practical utility of these measures. Instead, program leaders may want to survey practitioners directly to determine how acceptable a practice is to them. In general, direct questions (e.g., "Do you support the decision by your agency to adopt practice X?") are more useful than general attitudinal measures. Put simply, clinicians may have favorable attitudes toward one evidence-based practice while harboring negative attitudes toward another.

To illustrate this point, consider a widely used general attitudinal scale, the Evidence-Based Practice Attitude Scale (EBPAS) (Aarons 2004). It assesses general acceptability of evidence-based practices with a fifteen-item checklist completed by practitioners and program leaders. While the EBPAS is simple to administer and is intuitively appealing, it is limited to measuring global reactions to the concept of implementing evidence-based practices without regard to specific features of a particular practice, such as whether it requires the use of a treatment manual (Borntrager, Chorpita, Higa-McMillan, and Weisz 2009).

Practice's Acceptability to Clients

For an intervention to be successful, it must be acceptable to clients receiving it. Although client satisfaction ratings are widely used to monitor client acceptability, we caution against their use. Satisfaction surveys are often uninformative because mental health clients tend to show a strong bias toward rating their care favorably. A more direct approach is to measure actual behavior. For example, program leaders might track how frequently clients enroll in services when they are offered to them and how frequently they drop out of programs. In other words, low rates of enrollment and high dropout rates are direct indicators of poor client acceptability. (The enrollment rate described here refers to services that are readily accessible but that many clients show no interest in receiving.) The criteria for identifying dropouts and dropout rates vary widely and to some extent depend on characteristics of each evidence-based practice. For example, in practices with a fixed curriculum and fixed number of sessions, the dropout rate is usually defined as the number of participants who fail to attend a minimum number of sessions. For interventions that do not have fixed time limits or are conceptualized as "time unlimited," the dropout rate is usually defined as the percentage of participants who discontinue services within a prescribed short period of time, such as within six months after program admission.

Organizational Readiness

Many published general-purpose organizational scales are easy to administer and widely used in research, but they lack the specificity needed to guide an implementation effort. Because of their limited practical value, we do not recommend any such measures. Instead, we recommend using checklists tailored to specific evidence-based practices measuring an organization's readiness to implement a specific practice. Two such tools are as follows:

The AIMS Team-Building Tool is a detailed five-page self-assessment template that helps health care organizations identify the steps needed to implement a collaborative care program (AIMS Center 2011). Collaborative care, in this context, refers to a systematic approach to detecting and treating depression in primary care settings. Developed by the Advancing Integrated Mental Health Solutions Center, the AIMS Team-Building Tool helps organizations to identify resource gaps and staffing needs.

The Agency Readiness for IPS Supported Employment Checklist (Swanson and Becker 2011) serves as a guide to an initial consultation visit to a site. The twelve-item checklist is intended to pinpoint readiness issues around staff attitudes, leaders, and resources that will need to be addressed if implementation is to be successful.

Governmental/Funding Agency Leadership

The impetus to implement an evidence-based practice often comes from a state agency seeking to improve services throughout the state. Assessment tools have been developed to gauge the influence of state leadership. Similar to agency-level instruments used for quality improvement purposes at the service agency level, state agency assessment tools can be used to give feedback to state administrators for quality improvement purposes.

The State Health Authority Yardstick (SHAY) assesses the role of the state or government entity overseeing the services within a state or jurisdiction (Finnerty et al. 2009). This scale is a fifteen-item behaviorally anchored checklist designed to assess the presence of conditions associated with successful implementation of evidence-based practices in community mental health centers. It assesses the state mental health authority's role in seven domains: Planning, Financing, Training, Leadership, Policies and Regulations, Quality Improvement, and Stakeholders. Independent assessors complete the SHAY during a daylong site visit, interviewing key state leaders, examining policy documents, and reviewing other source material. The SHAY was originally developed for use with state mental health authorities, but it can be adapted for use with other state agencies responsible for treatment of substance abuse and other conditions.

Find the SHAY rating scale on the CD-ROM.

Indicators of Success: Implementation Measures

In the preceding section, we discussed factors that can impede or facilitate an implementation and the assessment tools for evaluating these factors. In this section, we consider outcomes that are direct indicators of the quality of an implementation. We'll examine five outcome domains—adoption, penetration, fidelity, model adaptation, and maintenance—and the tools for adequately assessing them.

Adoption

The Adoption Decision Factor Survey, developed by Panzano and Roth (2006), uses interviews with key program leaders to assess their beliefs and attitudes toward adopting an evidence-based practice. The survey instrument consists of forty-four items measuring eleven factors:

perceived risk, experiential evidence, scientific evidence, risk management capacity, ease of use, compatibility, knowledge set, dedicated resources, risk propensity, learning encouragement, and management's attitude. The authors have postulated that early adopters (that is, agencies that are the first to adopt an evidence-based practice) (Rogers 2003) would assess the risks of adopting as lower and would have a greater inclination to take risks than non-adopters (that is, agencies that do not adopt). A low score on this index would suggest caution in prematurely investing resources in staff training and implementation. In addition, the specific areas of concern on this index indicate areas for further discussion and education as a prelude to adoption.

Penetration

The degree of acceptance and participation in a program is often expressed as its penetration. We define a practice's penetration as the proportion among all eligible clients who are participating in a practice. It is expressed as the number of clients receiving an evidence-based practice divided by the total number of eligible clients in the population or agency. For example, in a dual disorders program located within a mental health center, the denominator would consist of the total number of clients at the center who have mental illness and a co-occurring substance use disorder.

Penetration is sometimes difficult to measure because of the difficulty of clearly identifying or quantifying a program's target population (what sometimes is called the "denominator problem"). An obvious challenge in measuring penetration is determining who meets the eligibility criteria. In addition, it is sometimes difficult to determine even the number receiving the services, owing to ambiguities about who is still an "active" client and whose file is closed. Nevertheless, we recommend including penetration as one implementation measure, because even if a program is highly effective, if clients cannot access it, its overall impact is diminished.

Fidelity

The most common standard for assessing the quality of an implementation is program fidelity. Fidelity refers to the degree to which a specific implementation adheres to the standards set in a program model. A fidelity measure is an instrument or method to measure program fidelity. The approach to measuring fidelity is guided in part by the nature of the intervention being evaluated. In psychotherapy, fidelity is typically measured at the practitioner or client level. The practitioner's skills and the client's outcomes are the focus of the evaluation. For team-based interventions, such as ACT and supported employment, a program-level fidelity scale is typically used. That is, several factors in the agency or program as a whole are assessed. Organizational-level fidelity scales are appropriate for practices requiring the shared efforts of staff throughout an organization and for practices that must be adopted across different departments and at different levels within the organization.

Practices can be classified as either curriculum based or action focused. Curriculum-based practices aim at imparting knowledge or teaching skills, while action-oriented practices are designed for clients to achieve macro-level functional outcomes, such as obtaining employment or independent housing. Fidelity scales for curriculum-based interventions typically track how many specific modules participants completed. For example, the curriculum-based intervention IMR consists of a series of sessions on specific topics such as identifying recovery goals and developing relapse prevention plans. Action-oriented practices, on the other hand, typically do not include the completion of discrete modules, and the fidelity scales for these evidence-based practices do not assess for completion of specific curricular content.

The methods for assessing practice fidelity also vary widely. In one approach, independent assessors interview staff, conduct chart reviews, and observe the program in action. A second type of fidelity review involves the coding of audiotaped or videotaped therapy sessions. A third involves checklists completed by practitioners, clients, or independent observers.

We offer this guideline: whenever feasible, independent assessors should observe programs directly rather than rely on self-report instruments. Independent observation avoids the biases that are associated with reports based on the opinions of program leaders, who are typically invested in "looking good." Another disadvantage of many self-report measures is that they use subjective rating scales. Such subjective tests may not be valid.

Whenever feasible, independent assessors should observe programs directly rather than rely on self-report instruments.

Based on our research in the National Implementing Evidence-Based Practices Project, we recommend using a specific structured approach to measuring fidelity for team-based evidence-based practices as listed in table 6. As part of this project, we developed implementation resource kits for five psychosocial practices highlighted in this book:

supported employment, ACT, IDDT, IMR, and family psychoeducation. Each of these kits includes a fidelity scale (McHugo et al. 2007).

The National Implementing Evidence-Based Practices Project fidelity scales share a common conceptual and methodological framework. All are multi-item scales derived from a set of core principles defining the practice. Items are rated by independent assessors using multiple sources of observation during the course of a site visit. Each item is rated on a five-point scale, with each scale point defined by observable criteria. A score of 5 indicates a high level of fidelity, and a score of 1 indicates a lack of fidelity, with intermediate scores representing gradations between low and high fidelity. A total score is calculated as the sum of the items. In the National Implementing Evidence-Based Practices Project, a site's average fidelity score (the total score divided by the number of items assessed) determined what level of program fidelity it had achieved. A site achieved a high-fidelity implementation if it had a score of at least 4. We have included three of these fidelity scales in their current, revised forms in the appendix: Supported Employment Fidelity Scale (2008, 2011), Dartmouth ACT Fidelity Scale, and Illness Management and Recovery Fidelity Scale.

Find the fidelity scales on the CD-ROM.

With the exception of general measures of quality of clinical care, each fidelity measure described in this chapter is by definition specific to an evidence-based practice. They include scales used to evaluate EBP implementation at the organization, program, and practitioner levels. All of these scales have "face validity"; that is, the measured items make sense in practical terms to clinicians. All have gone through a process of testing and refinement, and all have been used in either quality improvement or research applications or both. Most also have been studied for their capacity to measure change over time. Some of these measures show a positive correlation with external criteria, such as better client outcomes. All the scales listed in table 6 have our endorsement as being useful for either quality improvement or research applications, and most are useful for both purposes. But we also present these instruments as examples of the range of fidelity scales currently available and as models for developing scales tailored to other evidence-based practices.

Measures of Clinical Care

The General Organizational Index (GOI) is a general measure of the quality of clinical care implemented (Bond, Drake, Rapp, McHugo, and Xie 2009). The GOI consists of two five-item subscales: *Quality*

Improvement (training, supervision, process monitoring, outcome monitoring, and quality assurance) and *Individualization* (individualized eligibility determination, individualized assessment, individualized treatment plan, individualized treatments, and client choice). These scales were moderately correlated with EBP fidelity in one study.

The general approach to measurement is the same one used in the five EBP fidelity scales developed in the National Implementing Evidence-Based Practices Project. Independent assessors complete the GOI ratings during a site visit, typically in conjunction with fidelity assessments of a specific evidence-based practice. Because the ratings are made in reference to a specific practice, the GOI is not intended as a general-purpose scale. However, it could be adapted for general use in a service agency.

We next discuss three related *organizational*-level fidelity scales. In the next section, we discuss fidelity scales measuring evidence-based practices implemented at the *program* and *practitioner* levels.

The Dual Diagnosis Capability in Addiction Treatment (DDCAT) Version 4.0 index is a measure of an addiction treatment facility's organizational capacity to offer integrated substance abuse and mental health services (McGovern, Matzkin, and Giard 2007). It consists of thirty-five evaluated items in the following seven areas: Program Structure, Program Milieu, Clinical Process: Assessment, Clinical Process: Treatment, Continuity of Care, Staffing, and Training.

A comparable measure to the DDCAT, the Dual Diagnosis Capability in Mental Health Treatment (DDCMHT) Version 4.0 is an organizational index measuring the extent to which a mental health treatment program offers integrated substance abuse and mental health services (Gotham, Claus, Selig, and Homer 2010). It consists of thirty-five rated items grouped into the following seven subscales: Program Structure, Program Milieu, Clinical Process: Assessment, Clinical Process: Treatment, Continuity of Care, Staffing, and Training. Both indexes are designed to be completed during a site visit conducted by independent assessors.

The Dual Diagnosis Capability in Health Care Settings (DDCHCS) Version 2.0, based on a framework similar to the DDCAT and DDCMHT, is an organizational fidelity index measuring the extent to which both mental health and addiction treatment services are integrated into routine medical care settings such as primary care, federally qualified health centers, and family or pediatric practices. The index consists of

> Find the dual-diagnosis measures on the CD-ROM.

thirty-six items organized into the following seven subscales: Program Structure, Program Milieu, Clinical Process: Assessment, Clinical Process: Treatment, Continuity of Care, Staffing, and Training. The evaluation, like those for the DDCAT and DDCMHT, is conducted on site by independent assessors.

Fidelity Scales for Specific Practices

The Supported Employment Fidelity Scale (Becker, Swanson, Bond, and Merrens 2011) is an example of a program-level fidelity scale. Revised in 2008, it consists of twenty-five items, with each item reflecting a specific element in the practice. Items are rated on a five-point behaviorally anchored scale, with a rating of 5 indicating close adherence to the model and 1 representing substantial lack of model adherence. For example, the fidelity item Rapid Job Search is scored 5 if the first contact with an employer occurs on average within one month after the client enters the program, whereas programs where clients experience a delay of up to one year before they meet with a potential employer would receive a score of 1. Ratings of 4, 3, and 2 represent gradations between these two extremes.

Two trained fidelity assessors conduct the program evaluation using the Supported Employment Fidelity Scale, and the evaluations can be completed over the course of a day-and-a-half site visit. Assessors follow a detailed fidelity manual that provides instructions for preparing sites for the visit, describes critical elements in the fidelity assessment, and includes sample interview questions (Becker, Swanson, Bond, and Merrens 2011). The assessors interview program staff and clients, observe team meetings and community contacts with employers, and review client charts. After the site visit, each assessor independently makes fidelity ratings. The assessors then reconcile any discrepancies in their scoring to arrive at the final fidelity ratings. For quality improvement purposes, the assessors prepare a report summarizing the fidelity ratings and providing recommendations concerning any deficient components of the practice.

The Supported Employment Fidelity Scale is relatively easy to use and, in practice, results in an excellent agreement between the scores of independent assessors. The scale has been very well received as a quality-improvement tool, and high scores on the scale have been found in one study to correlate with competitive employment outcomes (Bond, Peterson, Becker, and Drake 2012).

The Dartmouth Assertive Community Treatment Scale (DACTS) (Teague, Bond, and Drake 1998) assesses fidelity to the ACT model. A twenty-eight-item program-level measure, the scale examines fidelity in three domains: Human Resources, Organizational Boundaries, and Nature of Services. Areas of inquiry within Human Resources include caseload ratio and the representation of specific professional disciplines and specialties on the team (e.g., nursing and psychiatry). Items covered under Organizational Boundaries include admission and discharge policies. The Nature of Services domain features queries on the intensity and location of services. The assessment and scoring procedures are similar to those used in the Supported Employment Fidelity Scale, and the fidelity assessment can be completed in one day.

The DACTS focuses on structural aspects of the ACT model. Most of the items are concrete and observable, and independent fidelity assessors generally agree on most ratings. The DACTS, either in its original form or in adapted form, has been used in hundreds of programs around the world. (The DACTS also appears in SAMHSA's ACT toolkit.)

The Tool for Measurement of Assertive Community Treatment (TMACT) Summary Scale (Monroe-DeVita, Teague, and Moser 2011) is a significant expansion and modification of the DACTS and was created in response to criticisms of the DACTS. The forty-seven-item scale consists of six subscales, or areas of evaluation: Operations and Structure, Core Team, Specialist Team, Core Practices, Evidence-Based Practices, and Person-Centered Planning and Practices. The TMACT differs from the DACTS in that it includes items measuring the specific responsibilities of practitioners and in its measurement of a program's orientation to recovery. The TMACT is also more sensitive to change than the DACTS. Because of its length, the TMACT assessment requires a site visit of up to two days to complete.

Find the TMACT on the CD-ROM.

Implementations of the IMR evidence-based practice are assessed with the IMR Fidelity Scale (Mueser, Gingerich, Bond, Campbell, and Williams 2005), a thirteen-item program-level scale last revised in 2005. It assesses both the implementation of specific evidence-based interventions within the program, such as cognitive-behavioral therapy and motivational interviewing, and structural and curriculum-based elements of the program, such as the number of sessions held or content modules covered. In addition to employing site visits, as do the other National Implementing Evidence-Based Practices Project scales, the

IMR Fidelity Scale relies heavily on the use of checklists completed at the end of each IMR session.

The Illness Management and Recovery Treatment Integrity Scale (IT-IS) (McGuire et al. 2012) is a companion measure for the IMR Fidelity Scale. It measures practitioner competence and consists of thirteen required items and three optional items that are rated by assessors using audiotape recordings of IMR sessions. The scale developers suggest that it can be used for research and quality-assurance purposes and as a tool for supervisory feedback.

The Independent Tape Rating Scale (ITRS) for Motivational Interviewing Fidelity Monitoring (Martino, Ball, Nich, Frankforter, and Carroll 2008) is another example of a fidelity scale measuring practitioner skills. Using audio-recorded counseling sessions, independent evaluators rate therapist interventions for adherence to and competence in motivational interviewing. The scale rates practitioners on five items reflecting fundamental skills, five items measuring advanced skills, and ten therapist actions deemed inconsistent with motivational interviewing.

The Yale Adherence and Competence Scale (YACS) assesses fidelity to the model of individual or group psychotherapy and skill in delivering the intervention. The YACS format provides specific adherence and competence measures for the most common behavioral therapies, including motivational interviewing, cognitive-behavioral therapy, interpersonal therapy, contingency management, and Twelve Step facilitation therapy. It also lays out a template for other behavioral therapies to be examined. The YACS and derivative scales are designed for ratings based on direct observation or audio-recorded or video-recorded review of actual therapy sessions (Carroll et al. 2000).

Alec Miller and colleagues developed a fidelity tool to assess best practices in the area of prescribing medications for people with schizophrenia. Initially labeled the MedMAP Fidelity Scale (Howard et al. 2009; Taylor et al. 2009), the terminology for the practice was changed to MedTEAM (Medication Treatment, Evaluation, and Management) (SAMHSA 2010). MedTEAM fidelity is assessed at both the prescriber and organizational levels. The organizational-level assessment is based on an interview and review of organizational forms and policies, while the prescriber-level assessment is based exclusively on client charts. MedTEAM is quite labor-intensive for paper records. Electronic medical

Find the fidelity tools on the CD-ROM.

records significantly shorten the time needed to complete the assessment (Tsai and Bond 2008).

Model Adaptation

Model adaptation refers to purposive modifications of an established EBP model. Adaptation is not identical with a lack of fidelity, although some model adaptations do result in reduced fidelity. Acceptable modifications to an evidence-based practice include additions to a model that do not compromise the practice's existing components. Examples of such additions might be incorporating a supported education component in a supported employment program or adding a peer counselor to the team providing an evidence-based practice when a peer counselor is not expressly specified in the original model. Some model adaptations may reflect realities of the setting. For example, in rural areas, daily team meetings required in the ACT model may not be practical. Still other acceptable adaptations can arise out of an agency's interest in responding to clients in a culturally appropriate way. New research findings may prompt other EBP modifications.

Maintenance

The measures in this section are especially useful for leaders involved in multi-site dissemination projects, such as learning collaboratives (Becker, Drake, Bond, Nawaz et al. 2011) and statewide initiatives. By collecting information on programs that have survived as well as those that have opted not to continue, program leaders can gain insight on strategies to achieve long-term success.

It is important not only to track the effectiveness of an implementation but also to assess how well a practice has been maintained. Maintenance of a practice, also referred to as *sustainability*, has proven to be an especially thorny construct to define in practical terms. One definition of sustainability in the research literature is "the extent to which a newly implemented treatment is maintained or institutionalized within a service setting's ongoing, stable operations" (Proctor et al. 2011). As a working definition, we suggest that a program has been maintained when it has achieved a high-fidelity implementation for at least six months after initial start-up and training has been completed. In other words, if a program has never been fully implemented (as measured by a fidelity scale), then it cannot be assessed for maintenance.

> A program has been maintained when it has achieved a high-fidelity implementation for at least six months.

Developed as a follow-up to the National Implementing Evidence-Based Practices Project, the Dartmouth Sustainability Interview allows reviewers to analyze the factors helping to maintain a practice. It is now being used in a subsequent project (Bond, McHugo, Becker et al. 2012). This semi-structured interview is to be conducted with program leaders and includes both open-ended questions (e.g., "Identify the three most important factors that have helped you continue your program") and Likert-type ratings on thirteen potential factors influencing sustainability. Follow-up interviews from the National Implementing Evidence-Based Practices Project found significant differences in factor ratings between sustainers and non-sustainers (Swain, Whitley, McHugo, and Drake 2010). The interview protocol could be adapted for use with other evidence-based practices.

The Decision to De-Adopt Index was assessed in a study examining factors leading to the discontinuation of a range of practices implemented as part of a statewide initiative (Massatti, Sweeney, Panzano, and Roth 2008). The researchers identified five indicators that an organization is likely to discontinue practice, which most often included a lack of financial resources and problems related to attracting and retaining qualified staff.

Putting It All Together

To truly understand the effectiveness of an implementation, you'll need to gather some data on the practice and its outcomes. In this section, we provide some specific suggestions for measuring a program's implementation and its results at your service agency. We also offer some guidance on how to improve the process of implementing and sustaining a new practice.

We begin with this recommendation on collecting data on your programs: *keep it simple*. As discussed earlier, data collection should be focused on specific key indicators and measures. The best indicators are those that are direct reflections of the intervention goals—competitive employment rates for supported employment, abstinence for IDDT programs, community tenure for supported housing—and those that reflect core principles of the evidence-based practice—frequency of employer contact for supported employment, percentage of home and community visits for ACT programs. Key indicators should make good sense to practitioners, program leaders, and external bodies. Ideally, key indicators are empirically supported by research attesting to their validity. Finally, key indicators are best when they have benchmarks showing performance levels in well-implemented programs (Becker, Drake, and Bond 2011).

Choosing appropriate measures is crucial. But it is not enough to simply measure something. This information must be shared with program staff and used to influence decision making. Nothing is more deadly than collecting data that are never examined. If the staff within an organization understand and believe that a set of specific measures is credible and important, then measurement is more likely to have an impact on implementation and ultimately on quality improvement.

Another reason to avoid excessive assessment of programs is its impact on data quality. When the burden on staff to collect data mounts, the care with which the data are recorded is often compromised. If too many measures are collected, then the focus will be diluted, and some measures will simply be ignored.

The scales, checklists, and other measures described in this chapter can, however, be brought together to assess the effectiveness of an implementation. Let's take the example of the evidence-based practice of supported employment. To measure organizational readiness, we recommend using the Agency Readiness for IPS Supported Employment Checklist (Swanson and Becker 2011). To measure agency-level penetration, you'll need to determine what percentage of clients is participating in the program. This can be calculated by dividing the number of clients receiving supported employment services by the total number of eligible clients in your agency who expressed an interest in receiving employment services. Often, however, you may not have data sources for estimating the number of eligible clients. If this is the case and you don't know the number of clients who have expressed a desire to work, then you can use a proxy percentage of 60 percent. (This number is based on research findings on supported employment.) The total number of clients with severe mental illness is multiplied by 60 percent to give the denominator in the penetration calculation.

Find the checklist on the CD-ROM.

To measure fidelity, we recommend using the Supported Employment Fidelity Scale (Becker, Swanson, Bond, and Merrens 2011). To track client outcomes, we recommend measuring the quarterly competitive employment rate among clients enrolled in supported employment (Becker, Drake, and Bond 2011). The quarterly competitive employment rate is calculated as the number of clients competitively employed (at least one day) divided by the number of clients active on the caseload during a ninety-day period.

Once Information Is Collected, What Should Be Done with It?

The purpose of collecting data from implementation measures is to improve services. But assessing practices and measuring outcomes is not enough. This information must be compiled in a usable form—that is, into a summary report—and shared with the relevant staff and other stakeholders. It is therefore incumbent on program leaders to not only judiciously collect the data of interest but also convert that raw data into a usable summary statement. It also is not sufficient to simply distribute summary reports without comment or follow-up. The most effective use of this data is in clinical supervision sessions in which staff are assessed on behaviors that they have the capacity to change. For example, we know that frequency of contact with employers is a key factor in determining the frequency of job starts. To improve outcomes, IPS supervisors can therefore monitor employment specialists on their rate of face-to-face contact with employers.

How Often Should an Implementation Be Measured?

Program leaders can better decide on how frequently to collect data on implementations after considering what kind of burden such data collection places on staff and how such data can be used in regular work routines. Measures that are relatively simple to collect and are routinely used in supervision should be collected on an ongoing basis. Employment rates, for example, can be generated from electronic medical records that track program admissions, terminations, and job starts. All three of these events should be recorded in real time. This information can then be summarized and compiled for occasions when you are most likely ready to review it, such as in supervision sessions.

When outcome measurement involves labor-intensive data collection, such as is the case with client questionnaires (which we do not recommend for most applications), data collection and reporting can be carried out less frequently. For example, for practical reasons, an IMR group leader might administer a self-report recovery scale to participants before enrollment in the course and then after the course has ended.

Fidelity assessments are more labor intensive. For team-based practices, we recommend that you conduct frequent fidelity assessments during the start-up phase of implementation, for example, at baseline, and then again at six and twelve months. Annual assessments are to be held during the latter part of the implementation stage. Once in the maintenance stage of implementation, fidelity assessments may taper off or be abbreviated as long as the program maintains good outcomes.

How frequently you should conduct fidelity assessments will be determined in part by the resources you have to conduct the measures. As information technology improves, practitioners can expect an increased use of electronic records, and these records may likely serve as the primary repository for most fidelity data. Electronic data collection and reporting should make it easier to track outcomes and assess how well an evidence-based practice has been implemented. But a certain amount of clinical judgment is required for some items on most fidelity scales. Data collection on such fidelity items is less easily automated.

How frequently you will need to conduct fidelity assessment of practitioner interventions will be guided by the time practitioners require to achieve competency. Once that phase has ended, fidelity checks are needed less frequently.

Other Uses of Implementation Measures

For agencies, implementation measures can help facilitate the implementation of an evidence-based practice and promote continuous quality improvement. But implementation measures can also be used in the context of formal research studies, multi-site dissemination projects, and program accreditation efforts.

Research studies use fidelity measures to ensure that the programs being evaluated are in fact implemented as intended. Journals now require researchers to report fidelity ratings for programs so that readers can evaluate how credible study findings are.

Multi-site dissemination projects include state-agency initiatives to implement evidence-based practices on a wide scale. State planners are interested in high-quality implementations of evidence-based practices and seeing that these standards are maintained in the long term. To help providers reach these goals, state agencies may require that participating provider agencies meet the practice criteria set by fidelity scales or other performance standards. Dissemination has also occurred at the national level. The Department of Veterans Affairs has led a number of national EBP initiatives (Resnick and Rosenheck 2009), as have several other federal agencies (Frey et al. 2011).

State agencies often provide financial incentives for attaining high-fidelity implementation. For example, in several states, employment programs achieving a benchmark on the Supported Employment Fidelity Scale receive a higher rate of reimbursement for services. Similarly, some states have an accreditation process for ACT. Case management programs that are accredited as ACT programs are reimbursed at a higher rate than are those case management programs not meeting this standard.

Summary

Measuring an implementation is a critical ingredient in identifying and achieving a successful program implementation. Program data can provide the best information on performance, and when approached pragmatically, assessment can provide information that is likely to lead to positive change. In this chapter, we have recommended a number of measures for use with specific evidence-based practices. In addition, we have identified several important aspects of a practice that should be considered but for which we do not at present have valid measures. It is our hope that agency leaders make use of these existing measures to quantify processes and outcomes and improve services.

3

The Checklist Approach to Implementation: Who Needs to Do What When

LIKE ATUL GAWANDE, author of *The Checklist Manifesto,* we appreciate the competing and sometimes overwhelming volume of decisions that professionals need to make in everyday practice situations. Gawande, a Boston surgeon, observed the benefits of using a simple checklist in the operating room and discovered that other professionals from airline pilots to structural engineers have also benefited from using a helpful recipe of steps to ensure that things happen as designed. We similarly have found checklists to be useful. In this chapter, we identify the tasks that help ensure effective implementation, grouping them by role and by stage of implementation. These tasks are provided in a practical checklist format. (The checklists are available as downloadable documents on the CD-ROM.)

Research studies present several theoretical frameworks for conceptualizing the sequence, duration, dynamics, and significance of stages in the process of implementing an evidence-based practice. Based on our collective experience in implementing evidence-based practices and work in implementation science, we believe a three-stage model to be the most practical. As discussed in chapter 1, the three stages are preparation, implementation, and maintenance.

Critical roles are

- federal government agencies
- state regulatory agencies
- technical assistance center
- CEO of the treatment provider agency
- clinical director of the treatment provider agency

- team leader or clinical supervisor of the treatment provider agency
- practitioners (clinicians, counselors, case managers) of the treatment provider agency
- consumers of services (clients and family members)

In this chapter, we will consider the important tasks taken on by each of these participants in the implementation of an evidence-based practice.

Gawande in his book presents more of a concrete "to do" list. One can check an item off and then move on to the next. The tasks on the implementation checklists are more complex. They will require ongoing attention and may need to be refined with use in a real-world setting. Much like other complex behaviors (for example, parenting), few specific activities can get checked off and never returned to again.

> The tasks on the implementation checklists are more complex. They will require ongoing attention.

This chapter is organized by implementation roles and by the tasks required at each stage of implementation. We begin with the role of the federal authorities and proceed to the front lines of the clinical intervention. This approach in no way reflects a hierarchy of importance. In reality, the last group we discuss—clients and significant others, the consumers of health care services—have by far the most important and potentially influential role. Arming clients with information about evidence-based treatments can raise clients' expectations about their care and public demand for these practices. Public awareness of the benefits of evidence-based practices will likely create political and economic pressure on the health care delivery system. Clients can begin to demand information on outcomes and demand providers offer treatments with known effectiveness. Treatment providers can demand support and incentives for offering effective treatments from funders and payers. Developers of new treatments designed to become evidence-based practices must take into account client demands, as well as provider capacity and workforce fit. Funders will encourage the provision of effective treatments by incentivizing treatment providers and supporting their clients' requests for the best care possible. We see these as good outcomes.

The checklists describe the tasks of individuals serving in each specified role. The preparation checklists speak to the tasks that should be completed before the launch of the implementation. At the preparation stage, a meeting among all stakeholders to review the checklists can serve multiple purposes, including generating enthusiasm, clarifying expectations and responsibilities, and providing a road map for the process of implementation.

Implementation checklists should be completed at quarterly intervals during the first two years of active implementation. Much like the checklist's role in a pre-implementation meeting, the implementation stage checklists can also serve as the basis for discussion, rewarding positive steps, and troubleshooting problems.

Checklists at the maintenance stage should be completed near the end of the two-year active implementation period. Maintenance checklists outline the tasks that stand to sustain the practice over the long haul.

Role Area: Federal Government

In the United States, many federal government agencies support and promote the availability of behavioral health care, but the main ones are the Department of Health and Human Services Substance Abuse and Mental Health Services Administration (SAMHSA), including the Center for Substance Abuse Treatment (CSAT) and Center for Mental Health Services (CMHS) and the Rehabilitation Services Administration. Another U.S. federal government agency involved in behavioral health services, largely in a funding capacity, is the Centers for Medicare and Medicaid Services (CMS). With health care reform impending, the responsibility of the Health Resources and Services Administration (HRSA) could expand to include behavioral health within the context of traditional physical health or medical care service delivery. In other countries, the federal government may be less fragmented and in better position to take more active roles in the implementation of effective treatments and services.

In the checklist on pages 54–55, we consider the minimum role of a federal government to be its power to regulate service delivery (ensuring the safety, adequacy, and equality of care). We do not consider the potentially significant role, although critical, that the U.S. government plays in research funding, particularly through the National Institutes for Health (NIH). NIH can be instrumental in supporting implementation science research and fostering the discovery of evidence-based strategies to bridge the gap between what is known and what is practiced in routine health care settings.

Find the checklists on the CD-ROM.

The checklists for federal and state agencies recognize the critical role they can play in shaping regulations and public insurance support for evidence-based treatments and quality care.

PREPARATION STAGE

☐ Show tangible support by allocating resources or incentives

☐ Make public statements, produce documents, and provide conferences, webinars, and web-based resources

☐ Compile the evidence on evidence-based practices (literature reviews, meta-analyses, expert panels)

☐ Disseminate evidence in usable form for states and treatment providers (manuals, toolkits, treatment improvement protocols)

☐ Prioritize evidence-based practices in directives, rules, and policies

☐ Fund practices that are proven to be effective

☐ Eliminate funding for practices that are ineffective

IMPLEMENTATION STAGE

☐ Communicate with other government offices and publicly recognize programs engaged in implementing the practice

☐ Simplify rules for accessing funding for implementing evidence-based practices

☐ Establish conferences, webcasts, and learning communities as a means to provide mechanisms for mutual learning and problem solving

☐ Develop a mechanism for assessing state and program-level outcomes on penetration

☐ Generate aggregate reports on program and client outcomes using uniform data gathered from funded programs

☐ Develop professional and client directories of programs that have documented successful delivery of evidence-based practices

☐ Support and evaluate technical assistance centers on effective implementation of evidence-based practices

MAINTENANCE STAGE

☐ Continue to communicate with other governmental offices through public service announcements and awards to programs engaged in sustaining implementation efforts

☐ Build in mechanisms to ensure permanence and predictability in funding, such as through block grant mechanisms or federal health care reimbursement mechanisms

☐ Continue to provide mechanisms for relaying updates and new developments for mutual learning and problem solving through conferences, webcasts, and learning communities

☐ Continue gathering and reporting program-level outcome data on penetration

☐ Continue to create aggregate reports on program and client outcomes

☐ Maintain and update professional and client directories of programs that have documented successful delivery of evidence-based practices

☐ Continue to support and evaluate technical assistance centers on effective implementation of evidence-based practices and help the centers revise and update information based on the latest evidence

Role Area: State Government

In the United States, state governments assume the responsibility for overseeing the establishment of many public services, including health, safety, transportation, and education programs, as well as managing professional licensure and certification. Accordingly, state authority is substantial. States vary in the extent of their commitment to health care in general and behavioral health in particular. Nonetheless, in our experience, the state agency charged with the regulation of public health and/or behavioral health care is critical to ensuring effective implementation. These state agencies range from departments to divisions to offices. The respective leaders can be commissioners, directors, deputy directors, or coordinators. Behavioral health may be integrated with health or public health, separated, and/or divided into mental health and addiction services. There may be excellent alignment across the various departments, divisions, or offices, or there may be conflict among them or benign disinterest. Leaders can be short-term political appointees to lifelong public servants.

Several national organizations act to bring together state agency leadership. Among these are, for example, the National Association of State Mental Health Program Directors, the National Association of State Alcohol/Drug Abuse Directors, the National Academy for State Health Policy, and the National Association of State Medicaid Directors. Membership in these organizations is voluntary, but each group has potential to leverage widespread cultural, policy, and practice changes.

State authorities typically take on active regulatory functions to ensure public safety. An agency's accessibility; its adherence to laws and regulations relating to fire safety, client confidentiality, and record keeping; and its compliance with state regulations and policy are verified via official site visits. The state may require funded programs to be licensed, certified, or accredited. In addition, funding via federal block grants (such as funding through CSAT or CMHS) is transferred through state agencies. Private insurance claim payments may also be regulated through the state insurance authority.

Certain professions, such as those in medicine, psychology, social work, and counseling, as well as peer recovery programs, are also regulated through state licensing boards. These boards grant initial licenses and provide re-certification for existing licenses. Boards can be influenced by state leadership but have as their primary mission the protection of the public in services delivered by professionals in the regulated fields.

In general, states have considerable authority and are in a critical position to foster or inhibit the successful implementation of evidence-based practices. Via regulatory, licensing, certifying, funding, and leadership functions, the state's potential for good is enormous. The state's role at each stage of practice implementation can be described as follows:

PREPARATION STAGE

☐ Verbalize and demonstrate stable, long-term, positive commitment to implementing evidence-based practices

☐ Give key state agency staff the responsibility for implementing evidence-based practices

- ☐ Identify and provide funding for training, technical assistance, and implementation support

- ☐ Obtain all necessary materials (curriculum, manuals) for evidence-based practices

- ☐ Secure high-quality training and implementation support

- ☐ Identify mechanisms to track fidelity and adherence to program models and link with service and client-level outcomes

- ☐ Provide means to fund or create incentives for the delivery of evidence-based practices

IMPLEMENTATION STAGE

- ☐ Visit sites to communicate enthusiasm and commitment and to eliminate potential state system barriers

- ☐ Provide funding for training and consultation, including release time for agency leadership and clinical staff

- ☐ Train appropriate agency personnel in the evidence-based practice and use of all related materials and tools (focusing on training middle managers and/or clinical supervisors)

- ☐ Initiate fidelity and adherence monitoring, with data collection and feedback on service and client-level outcomes

- ☐ Ensure there is adequate funding or reimbursement for the evidence-based practice

- ☐ Monitor technical assistance and interagency learning communities

- ☐ Report findings to treatment-provider agency leadership and recognize and reward successful programs

MAINTENANCE STAGE

- ☐ Revise policies and regulations to support sustainability and ongoing implementation of the evidence-based practice

- ☐ Ensure ongoing opportunities for training and technical assistance (supervision) for new staff members

- ☐ Facilitate interagency learning communities and support leadership or master implementers

☐ Fund the delivery of the evidence-based practice

☐ Incorporate continuing fidelity or adherence monitoring into routine regulatory site visits, if possible

☐ Share service and client outcome data

☐ Use website and resource directories to share information about the availability of evidence-based services and to enhance public awareness

Role Area: Technical Assistance Center

Technical assistance centers are independent entities designed to bridge the gap between research and practice. Technical assistance centers typically employ either active or former clinical practitioners who are well versed in the real-world challenges of the work. These individuals, called consultants, coaches, or experts, also have extensive knowledge of effectiveness and services research as well as findings from implementation science. Given the unique expertise required of technical assistance centers, they are often based in academic centers. Some also have federal funding to "transfer technology" into routine community settings. The regional centers of the SAMHSA-funded Addiction Technology Transfer Center (ATTC) Network are an example. The Center for Evidence-Based Practices at Case Western Reserve University or our own research center, the Dartmouth Psychiatric Research Center, are examples of technical assistance centers housed in academic settings.

Technical assistance centers support the work of treatment providers and state agencies but lend a focus and expertise that the state agency itself typically cannot provide. The state agency relies on the technical assistance center to (1) maintain an up-to-date knowledge of and expertise in new and existing evidence-based practices; (2) present current, effective implementation strategies; (3) bring outside and objective credibility (recognizing the saying, "No prophet is honored in his own land"); and (4) bring an understanding of the implementation process and set realistic expectations.

Many states have ongoing relationships with technical assistance centers and support core operations through ongoing contracts. Other technical assistance centers are brought in to execute certain objectives on a project- or grant-specific basis. Some technical assistance centers serve a regional or national network of states and providers, whereas others are dedicated to a specific region.

Many technical assistance centers are developing expertise in implementation itself, allowing them to provide assistance on implementing a broad range of evidence-based practices. Other technical assistance centers are specialized, either by intervention (e.g., cognitive-behavioral therapy) or population (e.g., persons with severe mental illnesses).

Aside from the regional ATTCs, which have a national office, technical assistance centers are not bound together by any specific organizational or professional society. At the same time, many technical assistance centers are active in research programs and are engaged in both developing and disseminating practices.

As the emerging science of implementation begins to document the effectiveness of specific implementation strategies, technical assistance centers may need to work together more systematically.

Meanwhile, technical assistance centers continue to play an important role in implementation and have the following tasks:

PREPARATION STAGE

- ☐ Engage agencies in leadership (implementation) committees
- ☐ Ensure that site leadership is familiar with evidence-based practice
- ☐ Develop scope of work, including planned duration of involvement and implementation outcomes
- ☐ Consult with agencies on steps to prepare for and to implement evidence-based practice
- ☐ Prepare agencies for training and organize all materials (e.g., curriculum, PowerPoint presentations, handouts, forms)
- ☐ Ensure readiness for fidelity assessment and outcome monitoring by securing appropriate measures and procedures for data collection
- ☐ Lay groundwork for a learning collaborative, including facilitator, membership, frequency of meetings, and goals

IMPLEMENTATION STAGE

- ☐ Conduct skills-focused training on the evidence-based practice for agencies and providers

- ☐ Conduct pre-implementation or early implementation fidelity assessments

- ☐ Install systems to track pre-implementation or early implementation client or process outcomes

- ☐ Identify, train, and support implementation monitors and champions, team leaders, or clinical supervisors of the practice for troubleshooting problems

- ☐ Be available—whether onsite or through video- or teleconferencing—to troubleshoot, adapt, and/or refine the implementation

- ☐ Organize learning communities and support regular meetings and cross-site learning

- ☐ Identify high-performing sites for recognition and awards and encourage other agencies to visit and observe these sites

MAINTENANCE STAGE

- ☐ Clarify mechanisms for ongoing contact between the technical assistance center and agencies

- ☐ Establish a train-the-trainer model to continue implementation and train new hires

- ☐ Provide consultation for persistent or novel implementation challenges

- ☐ Train state or other agency to continue fidelity checks and provide detailed reports with target or goal fidelity ratings

- ☐ Support state, agency, and client efforts to sustain implementation with funding

- ☐ Shift leadership of learning collaborative to state or agencies

- ☐ Link state leaders with a larger community of other states or systems involved in maintaining and refining the practice

Role Area: Chief Executive Officer, Treatment Provider Agency

The chief executive officer or CEO of a treatment provider agency plays a key role in the success or failure of an implementation. The CEO cannot be neutral. Laissez-faire or hands-off approaches will doom the implementation process. The CEO must be visionary and inspirational but also needs to hold people accountable for the implementation. This may involve publicly supporting if not hailing the importance of the evidence-based practice. If the mission of the agency is client care, there should be no difficulty in offering this level of support and leadership.

The CEO is typically the nexus of multiple stakeholders: a board of directors, the state agency, community leaders, senior agency leadership, and clients and families. Leadership and diplomacy skills are essential. The CEO can bridge all of these stakeholders, if not galvanize them, in pursuit of a common goal of improving the prospects for recovery among the people the agency serves.

In selecting an evidence-based practice for implementation, the CEO has the responsibility to convince all stakeholders that the practice is worthwhile, if not essential, for excellent client care. Obtaining and maintaining this kind of belief and commitment in the practice's implementation over the long haul will go far to ensure its success. Communicating this message is crucial.

The CEO must consider completing the following tasks:

PREPARATION STAGE

- ☐ Go on record supporting the practice and enthusiastically noting how it is consistent with the mission of the agency
- ☐ Meet with stakeholders as a group and individually to discuss the evidence-based practice
- ☐ Identify potential barriers to implementation and strategies to overcome them
- ☐ Assign leadership roles and responsibilities within the agency
- ☐ Establish reporting pathways and chains of command and hold staff accountable
- ☐ Align medical records with the evidence-based practice, such as with specific prompts and headings
- ☐ Align funding with the evidence-based practice

IMPLEMENTATION STAGE

- ☐ Review progress on implementation with agency leaders and address deviations from the timetable to implement

- [ ] Oversee problem solving with active and regular monitoring
- [ ] Establish methods and practices to integrate the evidence-based practice with existing clinical operations, workflow, and staff responsibilities
- [ ] Recognize and affirm success
- [ ] Connect with other agency CEOs implementing the evidence-based practice
- [ ] Attend learning community sessions for senior leadership
- [ ] Demand agency data on the relationship between the evidence-based practice and client and process outcomes

MAINTENANCE STAGE

- [ ] Reiterate, in public and agency meetings, the agency's long-term commitment to sustaining the evidence-based practice
- [ ] Continue to monitor reports on program fidelity and client and process outcomes
- [ ] Empower clinical leaders to make decisions and take action
- [ ] Ensure financial and policy support for the practice
- [ ] Reward successful team leaders and staff members
- [ ] Ensure that staff can maintain an ongoing high-quality practice: hire, fire, transfer as necessary
- [ ] Support participation of senior leaders or clinical supervisors in learning communities to keep up to date on practice and materials

Role Area: Clinical Director, Treatment Provider Agency

An agency's clinical director may be the individual most knowledgeable about the agency's prospects for successfully implementing any given evidence-based practice. Either through analyzing the data or by anecdote, the clinical director may have some idea about staff attitudes, knowledge, and skill level. Directors may see the practice to be a logical and easy "fit" or a very difficult if not culture-changing one. They may consider how to select an evidence-based practice or may prioritize, integrate, or even critique the implementation of a new practice into the existing clinical operations.

Clinical directors must be able to distinguish between their own attitudes toward innovation and the opportunity for change versus the perceptions of staff. There are clinical directors who may be less open to evolution in the field and have firm ideas about tradition and what is correct. The entire field of implementation rests on the assumption that health care is constantly evolving, and it relies on clinical leaders who view these changes as being generally for the better in terms of client care and benefit. Thus, at a minimum, the clinical director must be open minded.

Of course, effective implementation is most likely when clinical directors are strong and passionate advocates for the evidence-based practice. They can be vocal and knowledgeable in conveying the importance to the practice in the clinical mission. They can demonstrate leadership and commitment by figuring out who are the most capable supervisors and clinicians to catalyze the implementation. They can be the clinical administrator in charge of how the rollout will occur, how the implementation will be monitored, how meetings will take place, and by what agenda meetings will be guided. They will influence how the practice will be integrated into routine operations down the road. The role of the clinical director is critical, and the director's tasks are as follows:

PREPARATION STAGE

- [ ] Know about the evidence for the practice and the realities of implementation to "sell" to the CEO and clinical leaders
- [ ] Plan how the practice will fit into existing scheduling, workflow, and staff capacities
- [ ] Initiate or modify existing policies so that they are consistent with the implemented evidence-based practice
- [ ] Plan and oversee training and coordinate consultation and ongoing support received from the technical assistance center
- [ ] Identify and work with capable team leaders and champions for the implementation
- [ ] Form an implementation task force or work group and meet on a regular basis
- [ ] Plan how to incorporate fidelity, benchmark measures, or adherence/ competence monitoring into routine clinical supervision or quality improvement department activities

☐ Locate a learning community that can provide support for the implementation

IMPLEMENTATION STAGE

☐ Ensure that appropriate skill-based training in the practice occurs and that relevant staff members are exposed to the practice

☐ Make use of a technical assistance center to work on organizational changes and on ongoing support and supervision

☐ Ensure that fidelity, benchmark, or adherence/competence monitoring is in place and linked with client and process outcomes

☐ Support new practice leaders with staff and workflow changes

☐ Meet with the task force or work group to troubleshoot barriers/challenges to the implementation

☐ Align policy with practice and minimize any additional paperwork or workload

☐ Attend learning community meetings as an agency representative

MAINTENANCE STAGE

☐ Secure the place of the evidence-based practice on the program schedule and routine workflow

☐ Ensure that policy support for the evidence-based practice is documented

☐ Integrate fidelity, benchmark, or adherence/competence monitoring into routine agency operations, including clinical supervision, case review, team meetings, medical record keeping, or quality improvement procedures

☐ Recognize and reward high achievers in the implementation

☐ Improve the consistency with which the practice is implemented across the agency

☐ Maintain ongoing meetings among the implementation work group or task force members. Focus meeting discussions on sustaining the practice (training new staff, advanced practice issues, adaptations).

☐ Continue to participate in the learning community available through the technical assistance center

Role Area: Team Leader or Clinical Supervisor, Treatment Provider Agency

The agency team leader or clinical supervisor is typically charged with clinical practice at the program level. Agencies may have multiple programs, and the clinical director may have administrative responsibility for all programs across the agency. However, it is the team leader or clinical supervisor who is responsible for establishing a more-focused clinical service that might be delivered within a treatment program or by a specialized team that cuts across multiple programs within the agency. The team leader or clinical supervisor is clearly more in the "front line" and engaged in client care. Team leaders are most often either delivering services directly or engaged in individual or group supervision of the staff treating the client or delivering the practice. It is the team leader or clinical supervisor who is most key and most directly responsible for translating the evidence-based practice from theory into the reality of the clinical setting. It is the team leader or supervisor who is most likely to wrestle with the practice's "fit" in the agency—how it might be integrated into the setting and its practitioners' attitudes, knowledge, and skill levels. This person will have a good sense of the clinicians who are likely to embrace the new practice or who are likely to reject it. The team leader or clinical supervisor will also consider practical matters such as the time needed to train facilitators and integrate the practice into everyday work and discourse and how the higher-ups will evaluate work in the practice. Team leaders or clinical supervisors suffer the liabilities and reap the benefits of being part of "middle management" in the health care system.

Nonetheless, frontline practitioners implementing the evidence-based practice will look to the team leader or clinical supervisor to evaluate the practice. They may draw their observations from tracking behaviors, emotions, or attitudes of agency leaders. The practitioner's first question often is, "What does the team leader or clinical supervisor *really* think about this?" The second question is, "Is this something that will pass or is it here to stay?"

Clearly what the team leader or clinical supervisor really believes about the evidence-based practice will be pivotal to the success or failure of the practice's implementation. The individual in this position serves as the interface between agency administration and frontline providers: the middle manager. Enthusiasm or negativity about the implementation can influence the positive attitude of the practitioners and also

> What the team leader really believes about the evidence-based practice will be pivotal to the success or failure of its implementation.

undermine any new initiative. Qualitative studies on potential barriers or facilitating factors in effective and sustained practice implementation often find that it is the team leader or clinical supervisor who is key to the implementation's success.

An agency may have multiple clinical supervisors or team leaders. Not all may be identified by the CEO or clinical director to take the lead on an implementation project. If you have been selected to be a team leader or clinical supervisor, you've likely been chosen because you are perceived to be a person who can make new and important things happen. In most cases, being selected for this role is a very good sign.

The team leader or clinical supervisor has certain tasks in each step of an implementation.

PREPARATION STAGE

- ☐ Verify that you and key practitioners will receive expert and adequate skill-based training in the evidence-based practice
- ☐ Verify that all necessary support materials to deliver the practice are accessible and transferable to your clinical situation and setting
- ☐ Ensure that there is a learning community of other team leaders or clinical supervisors and that you are a member
- ☐ Provide feedback to the clinical director on how the agency workflow, policies and procedures, and staff expertise support or hinder implementation of the evidence-based practice
- ☐ Participate and have a clear role on the implementation task force or work group
- ☐ Know how the implementation is being measured and evaluated: through fidelity, benchmark, or adherence/competence assessments, and/or client and process outcomes
- ☐ Consider how to incorporate the measures into clinical supervision, team meetings, case review, record keeping, staff evaluation, and routine new staff orientation and existing staff in-service training

IMPLEMENTATION STAGE

- ☐ Participate in training and ensure that all relevant staff are trained

- ☐ Work with the technical assistance center to identify the tasks for each implementer's role and utilize appropriate forms to evaluate practice implementation and client outcomes
- ☐ Discuss cases and review implementation and client outcomes as a team
- ☐ Document practice delivery and client response in records
- ☐ Use direct observation methods to supervise staff
- ☐ Work with practitioners who are struggling and draw on the technical assistance center's support in these efforts
- ☐ Attend learning community meetings to discuss challenges and learn from other team leaders and clinical supervisors' experiences

MAINTENANCE STAGE

- ☐ Continue using direct observational methods in providing clinical supervision
- ☐ Incorporate practice monitoring into your regular supervision, team meetings, and staff evaluation using fidelity, benchmark, or adherence/competence ratings
- ☐ Incorporate client- and process-outcome monitoring into regular supervision, team meetings, and staff evaluation
- ☐ Reward high-performing practitioners
- ☐ With help from a technical assistance center, find and support opportunities for practitioners to engage in learning communities or advanced "master" clinician circles
- ☐ Participate in an agency work group or task force to sustain the practice
- ☐ Make sure that new staff receive training and that existing staff have periodic in-service updates

Role Area: Practitioner, Clinician, or Counselor, Treatment Provider Agency

In many respects, the practitioner embodies the implementation. Often it is the individual in this role who is being asked to change the most. As we know from our efforts to help clients, change can be difficult.

Everyone has a firm connection to what they already do. It's the scientific principle of homeostasis at work.

Sometimes, however, problems with new initiatives happen at the organizational level. Practitioners may feel that they are at the bottom of the decision-making chain. At times, they may feel that decisions or mandates on new practices come down from the top without any practical consideration, let alone input, from those on the front lines. Practitioners may have experienced an impermanence or fluidity in management decisions and feel that in time the mandate will pass and things will return to normal.

In this chapter, we have attempted to consider implementation as an organization-wide activity. We have outlined the tasks required of the team leader or clinical supervisor, the clinical director of the agency, and the CEO. Successfully completing these tasks can help verify whether the evidence-based practice is a good fit for the agency and setting. The supports outlined in these tasks should help ensure that practitioners are well prepared to learn and deliver the new practice. To encourage acceptance of the new practice, practitioners should be given the means and the opportunity to provide feedback and to suggest necessary adaptations based on their experience.

Even when all these conditions are met, the practitioner also has a job to do in the implementation process. In fact, this job is essential. Practitioners, clinicians, and counselors have the following tasks in the implementation process:

PREPARATION STAGE

- ☐ Stay open-minded to the change: consider ways the evidence-based practice can work and improve care
- ☐ Confirm that there is time and opportunity for training
- ☐ Understand how the practice will fit into your current schedule and workload
- ☐ Openly discuss practical concerns about implementing the practice to help management "think through" potential barriers
- ☐ Consider how or if the practice will affect the existing clinical practice, including specific clients
- ☐ Be clear about how the practice will be documented in the medical record and discussed in team meetings and supervision

☐ Insist that fidelity, benchmark, or adherence/competence assessments be transparent and that client outcomes be shared

IMPLEMENTATION STAGE

☐ Master the information and skills associated with the new evidence-based practice

☐ Use supervision and team meetings to discuss challenges and specific case issues

☐ Be patient and accept that any new practice requires repetition for practitioners to gain skills and comfort with it

☐ Be positive about the new practice when interacting with client and family members

☐ Challenge the policies, scheduling, workflow, and documentation procedures that interfere with efficiently delivering the new practice

☐ Directly observe team leaders or clinical supervisors working in the evidence-based practice

☐ Insist that data be collected on practice delivery, as well as client and process outcomes

MAINTENANCE STAGE

☐ Accept the practice as part of your everyday work routine

☐ Refine your knowledge and skill: work at getting better and more comfortable at delivering the practice

☐ Continue to request monitoring data from the supervisor, including fidelity assessments, adherence/competence ratings, and client and process outcomes

☐ To enhance your practical knowledge and skill, insist on having access to a learning community or "master" clinician group of peers

☐ Incorporate the practice into your routine schedule, workload, medical record keeping, case review, and clinical supervision

☐ Be positive and enthusiastic with new staff members about the practice

☐ Continue to use the practice when working with new and existing clients

Role Area: Clients and Families

Historically, the health care system has been hierarchical. The doctor had specialized knowledge and skill; the client did not. The client's "job" was to follow orders without question. "Non-compliant" was (and is) a term used to describe the client who did not follow orders.

Over the past decade, in part due to advances in medical science but also in part due to the heightened recognition of the centrality of the client, a more collaborative model of care has evolved. Although many health care providers and clients are uncertain about their roles in this model of care, it has demonstrable benefits. Clients and families who take a more active role in their care are (1) more satisfied with services, (2) more likely to engage in their treatment plan, and, perhaps not surprisingly, (3) have better outcomes.

Shared decision making is a health care strategy that sees the treatment provider as the expert in treatment options and the client as the expert in his or her disease experience and treatment preferences. This is an example of collaborative care. In shared decision making, an honest and empathic negotiation of preferences and options is emphasized and understood as the basis of the treatment provider-client relationship.

Informed clients are empowered stakeholders.

The public today has a tremendous amount of information about good and bad health care practices. Informed clients are empowered stakeholders. Access to better medical information means that clients and their families can demand adequate care, better access to care, and public and private insurance coverage. Clients have become a force to be reckoned with. We embrace this as a good development for the health care system.

As clients, their families, and significant others are informed about the value of evidence-based treatments, demand for their implementation increases. Client advocacy and consumer groups are increasingly aware of variations in quality of care across the health care marketplace. They are now approaching treatment providers and regulatory agencies with demands to address these discrepancies. Clients and families are increasingly playing a pivotal role in encouraging the implementation of evidence-based practices. Clients and their families can likewise play a pivotal role in ensuring that implemented evidence-based practices continue to be accessible and sustained over time. Clients can do the following:

PREPARATION STAGE

☐ Request information about practices that are based on evidence

☐ Advocate for the establishment of a client advisory board or request a representative on the agency's board of directors

☐ Advocate for a client voice in state government, including the offices that regulate health care

☐ Ask questions of treatment providers about access to evidence-based practices

☐ Talk publicly and to media outlets about the importance of evidence-based services

☐ Be supportive of other clients and families

IMPLEMENTATION STAGE

☐ Demand information about programs that do and do not use evidence-based practices

☐ Create a client's guide to services

☐ Demand information about the results of an agency's fidelity and/or benchmark assessments

☐ Demand information about the effectiveness of the evidence-based practices implemented at the agency. Are these programs being run as designed? What were the agency's findings on clients who participated in the practice? What impact did these programs have on their health?

☐ Participate regularly in advisory or client board meetings

☐ Enlist the support of other clients and family members

MAINTENANCE STAGE

☐ Demand that the state regulatory agency finance and support evidence-based practices

☐ Demand that the state regulatory agency make public a list of agencies offering evidence-based services that meet fidelity standards or benchmark measures

☐ Demand that the state regulatory agency make public an agency's client and process outcomes

☐ Continue to serve alongside treatment providers on boards and advocacy groups

☐ Stay informed of new developments—the field is constantly changing—and make use of the technical assistance center

Summary

In this chapter, we have detailed the specific tasks of each participant in the implementation process. Attention to these tasks ensures a successful implementation and the long-term sustainability of an evidence-based practice. The more tasks that are completed in each key role, the better the chances are for an effective implementation of the practice. (Remember, too, as practices evolve, they need continuing attention and problem solving and even adaptation. Everyone is responsible for working on improvements.)

Eight role areas have been described, with no more than seven checklist items at each stage of the implementation. You will find reproducible versions of the checklists on the CD-ROM that accompanies this book.

We encourage you to complete the checklist for your role and encourage others to complete the checklists for their roles as well. Assembling the team ahead of time and taking a good look at what is involved in the endeavor is an excellent strategy at the pre-implementation stage. The checklists can also serve to clarify expectations and provide a road map for the work that lies ahead.

4

Implementing Multiple Evidence-Based Practices Simultaneously

HEALTH CARE REFORM calls for health care services to become client-centered, integrated, multidisciplinary, team-based, evidence-based, and recovery-oriented. To approach this standard, behavioral health programs need to implement many evidence-based practices simultaneously. Yet program leaders and clinicians protest that they can implement only one new program at a time and that attaining high-fidelity implementation takes years. Implementing one practice at a time means, of course, that a system would never become evidence-based in any comprehensive sense. How can this tension be resolved?

Implementing one practice at a time, as has typically been done in research demonstration projects, is time-consuming and expensive. This approach focuses on helping one subgroup of clinicians learn these skills rapidly, often without involving other clinicians and without creating the infrastructure needed to support long-term maintenance of the practice. Too often, when the grant ends or the clinicians leave their posts, the evidence-based practice fades away.

Professionals in the behavioral health field must recognize that they aren't restricted to implementing one practice at a time with one group of clinicians. In fact, a few basic clinical skills constitute the building blocks for nearly all evidence-based practices. The essential underlying clinical skills include (1) motivational interviewing, (2) psychoeducation, (3) cognitive-behavioral interventions, and (4) community-integration interventions. As we shall show in this chapter, training in these skills can go a long way toward establishing a practice fully informed by evidence-based practices.

In real-world behavioral health programs, clinicians acquire and refine skills slowly as part of everyday clinical work and supervision. Most clinicians already have some level of basic skills and are eager to improve them. Thus, adopting the skills for evidence-based practices can be a natural transition.

With training, supervision, and program infrastructure in place, evidence-based practices can be implemented, monitored, and maintained over time. The key is providing the structures—the leadership, clinical supervision, record keeping, credentialing, and other processes—so that basic skills can be applied in different contexts and then sustained.

In this chapter, we first explain the fundamental building blocks that compose several evidence-based practices. We then discuss how these building blocks inform multiple evidence-based practices. Finally, we examine different stakeholders' perspectives on this process.

Basic Clinical Skills

Effective clinicians must be able to engage clients in the clinical work, assess their status and needs, educate them about potential interventions, collaborate with them to set goals, help them to achieve these goals by increasing their skills and enhancing their supports, and ensure success along the path to recovery. The key is that effective care is oriented to the client's perspective.

> Effective care is oriented to the client's perspective.

Clients are motivated to pursue their own goals and are reluctant to focus on their deficits. This reality has immediate implications. If clinicians start by identifying a list of problems to be addressed, clients tend to resist engagement, fearing that it will painfully reveal their wounds without enhancing their strengths. If, on the other hand, clinicians begin by identifying the client's skills and life goals and by helping to formulate plans to achieve those goals, clients become willing over time to acknowledge and address some of their problems. The clash in perspectives often reflects a divide between the emphasis on functional goals versus a focus on clinical symptom control. Clients typically prioritize functional goals, such as those related to housing or work. Clinicians typically prioritize symptom control, such as medication adherence or abstinence from substance use. Practitioners who cannot identify and address the client's functional goals will often fail to engage clients and ultimately fail to address illness management goals.

Let's consider an example of what effective care might look like. A young man with early schizophrenia, accompanied by his family, seeks help following a prolonged hospitalization. The clinical team meets with this young man and listens to his story, collects information from the hospital and family as well as from him, and provides education about schizophrenia and treatment options. The young client emphasizes his wish to return to school, to reconnect with his friends, and to reduce the medications he is taking because they cause extreme drowsiness. Assessment also indicates that his use of marijuana, association with friends who use marijuana daily, and disagreements with parents are problems, all of which he acknowledges. The treatment team and client agree on the following plan:

- Meet with the supported employment/education counselor to facilitate his returning to school with the supports he'll need to be successful.
- Join a group of other young people who are discussing their marijuana use.
- Meet with the team doctor to consider medication options.
- Meet with his family and a social worker to learn how to resolve disagreements.

The family endorses this plan and also agrees to attend local meetings of the family-to-family program. The team reviews these goals with the young man monthly and plots progress on the goals using simple scales. As the team and young man identify new goals, they add them to the list. The team members meet weekly to make certain they are working on the same plan and making progress.

After six months, the young man is enrolled in a community college and successfully completing two courses. He and his family have mastered basic information regarding schizophrenia and marijuana use. After several discussions with his doctor and reading articles, the young man is transitioning to a long-acting injectable medication that causes fewer side effects and eliminates the need to take medications each day. He is attending a young people's Alcoholics Anonymous group weekly with new friends. And the family has learned to address disagreements using a behavioral method to solve problems.

This scenario illustrates the essential, underlying clinical skills we introduced at the beginning of this chapter: (1) motivational interviewing, (2) psychoeducation, (3) cognitive-behavioral interventions, and (4) community-integration interventions. As a basic approach to the clinical encounter, motivational interviewing emphasizes the need to focus on and clarify what the client is saying, to prioritize the client's goals, to avoid conflict, and to help the client find step-wise solutions to achieve goals. Clinicians can use motivational interviewing in almost any situation. Psychoeducation refers to providing relevant information to enable the client (and the family) to understand the disorder and available interventions. Accurate information and intervention options inform shared decision making, which is sometimes called informed patient choice. Cognitive-behavioral interventions comprise a variety of techniques for helping clients examine and alter the thoughts that strongly affect their behaviors and to change behaviors in small steps. These strategies include functional analysis, cognitive restructuring, behavioral activation, self-monitoring, behavioral experiments, and relapse prevention. Community-integration interventions encompass techniques for helping the client find meaningful activities, learn skills, and make use of supports in the community. Natural supports may include friends, family, employment, religious affiliation, clubs, teams, and peer recovery support groups.

Most clinicians enter the job having these four skills in some degree. They may have learned skills in school and have probably tried to apply them in their practices. But the reality is that clinicians refine their skills over years in the context of doing clinical work and receiving supervision. The critical ingredient for such improvement is good supervision. Supervisors need to know these skills well, model them with supervisees, participate in practicing clinical scenarios, and observe actual clinical interactions. Effective supervision requires hands-on, field-based collaboration. In other words, professionals need coaches—clinicians need coaches as much as do athletes and musicians. Their skills will develop and improve through monitored and guided experience. Clinicians should increase their effectiveness over time, not repeat the same mistakes again and again. Good supervision is the key.

Basic Skills and Evidence-Based Practices

The four basic skills provide the foundation for evidence-based practices. If a clinician helps clients access and understand current information on behavioral disorders and effective treatments (that is, provides psychoeducation) and helps them select interventions and take ownership of treatment (or practices motivational interviewing), he or she is using these basic skills. If a clinician helps clients and their families learn new

Four basic skills provide the foundation for evidence-based practices.

coping strategies, the practitioner is employing the core skills of cognitive-behavioral treatment and family psychoeducation. If the clinician helps clients and families access natural supports through community-integration interventions and family psychoeducation, he or she is again using these basic skills. And if a clinician is helping the client to achieve personal recovery goals, he or she is using community-integration skills. These skills form the basis of evidence-based practices, and for each practice, these four skills can be blended into one coherent process.

Assertive community treatment (ACT) involves developing a trusting relationship with the client, educating the client regarding illness management and other potential interventions, enabling the client to identify his or her goals for community living, and helping the client to develop the skills and supports needed to attain those goals. Motivational interviewing establishes a trusting relationship and identifies goals. Illness management and recovery (IMR) and integrated dual disorders treatment (IDDT) include education, goal identification, and skill building. Supported education/employment builds supports for attaining school and employment goals. Family psychoeducation helps to build natural community supports. ACT cannot be provided without these clinical skills.

Table 7 shows the specific skills that underlie several common evidence-based practices, including ACT, illness/wellness management and recovery, supported employment/education, housing first, IDDT, family psychoeducation, and systematic medication management. Each evidence-based practice directs the skills in slightly different ways, as illustrated in table 7, but the basic building blocks are the same (see next page).

Using the Skills in an Evidence-Based Practice

Specialists who practice in a setting offering evidence-based practices may or may not have specific training in mental health or vocational services. But they must have the basic skills to provide psychoeducation, motivational interviewing, cognitive-behavioral interventions, and community-integration interventions. Let's take, for example, employment specialists. For this practice, these specialists must have the skills to facilitate community-integration interventions. The most critical aspect of their job description involves contacting employers to develop jobs that match clients' interests and skills. But employment specialists also need to educate clients about seeking and maintaining employment

TABLE 7
Basic Clinician Skills Used in Evidence-Based Practices

EVIDENCE-BASED PRACTICE	CLINICIAN SKILLS USED			
	Motivational Interviewing	Psychoeducation	Cognitive-Behavioral Interventions	Community-Integration Interventions
Assertive Community Treatment (Morse and McKasson 2005)	Setting and reevaluating goals	Explaining illness and alternative interventions	Developing skills for managing symptoms	Finding an apartment and a job
Cognitive-Behavioral Therapy*	Establish therapeutic alliance	Breathing retraining and symptoms of co-occurring disorders	Five steps of cognitive restructuring	Using cognitive-restructuring skills in peer recovery
Family Program*	Establish collaborative relationship with family	Educating families about co-occurring disorders and their treatment	Teaching families problem-solving and communication skills	Multiple family groups
Family Psychoeducation (Murray-Swank and Dixon 2005)	Establish collaborative relationship with family	Educating families about co-occurring disorders and their treatment	Teaching families problem-solving and communication skills	Refer family to National Alliance on Mental Illness
Housing First (Tsemberis 2010)	Help to choose housing	Housing basics: payments, landlords	Skills for managing housing	Outreach to client in apartment and to landlord
Illness Management and Recovery (Gingerich and Mueser 2011)	Establish personal recovery goals	Information and skills to assist in accomplishing personal goals	Role-plays, shaping, modeling, and home assignments to master skills and accomplish goals	Involving significant others to practice skills in the community
Integrated Dual Disorders Treatment (Fox, Drake, Mueser, Brunette et al. 2010)	Matching services to a person's readiness to change and stage of treatment	Understand how two disorders interact and the importance of integrating treatment	Relapse plans, social skills training, problem solving	Peer recovery support groups, work, supported housing, independent housing
IPS/Supported Employment (Swanson and Becker 2011)	Addressing ambivalence about working	Discussing the pros and cons of disclosure of psychiatric disability	Problem-solving conflicts and challenges in the workplace	Finding a job
Medication Management*	Choosing a medication	Understanding effects and side effects	Managing residual symptoms	Using coping skills in the community

*The practice as described in the Co-occurring Disorders Program. 2008. Center City, MN: Hazelden.

(psychoeducation), use motivational interviewing skills to assess their clients' interests and abilities, and draw on cognitive-behavioral interventions to help their clients adapt to the job. One leader who has these skills can train and oversee several employment specialists.

Specialists

Each practice involves a team, but it also relies on some clinicians becoming specialists. For example, within IDDT, one team member may work with families, one may provide educational groups, one may counsel clients directly, one may link clients with Alcoholics Anonymous and other support programs, and one may help clients to find jobs. If all clinicians have been working on the four basic skills, they will naturally gravitate toward one of these specialty roles. For example, clinicians who are in personal recovery will be more familiar with Twelve Step programs and may be able to link clients to these supports. Other clinicians will be drawn to educational groups because they are natural teachers or to community-integration in schools and jobs because they are naturally outgoing, and so on.

Take, for example, a program that provides residential care and ACT to people with co-occurring addiction and serious mental illness. This program developed specialists in exactly this way. All clinicians learned basic skills through training and supervision. One clinician with a background in family work began to work with the families, another who had worked in many businesses before pursuing a master's degree in counseling became an excellent supported education/employment specialist, another who enjoyed working with groups ran several dual recovery groups, and another in personal recovery became a liaison with Alcoholics Anonymous.

Sometimes the behavioral health program is starting a new team and can hire or transfer clinicians who already have the skills and experience for their roles. Several early psychosis teams have been constructed in this manner. For example, an early psychosis program hired a team leader with extensive supervisory experience, a behavioral skills trainer with cognitive-behavioral training, and an experienced supported education/employment specialist. These clinicians needed to learn basic skills and to work together, but they came prepared for their respective roles and coalesced as an effective team quickly.

Another program, a comprehensive addiction treatment agency, included residential, intensive outpatient, and outpatient services as well as drug court and methadone maintenance program components.

The agency trained all counselors, new and old, in the basic skills of motivational interviewing and cognitive-behavioral interventions. Supervisors participated in ongoing clinical supervision groups with experts from a technical assistance center, and supervision was carried out through direct observation, through using audiotapes, or through visiting group counseling sessions. Counselors and supervisors also used adherence and competence rating scales to evaluate performance and to improve skills.

Medical care is, of course, a highly specialized role. The medical specialist on the team, usually a nurse or doctor, must have medical training, but otherwise this specialist should be considered like other members of the team. Integrated care requires that the medical specialist understand what the entire team is doing and possess the same basic clinical skills. The medical specialist should be comfortable with psychoeducation, motivational interviewing, cognitive-behavioral interventions, and community-integration interventions. For example, the medical specialist should understand clients' goals, meet with families, endorse clients' motivation to work, and reinforce skills. Otherwise, having team members who do not employ these practices will cause mixed messages and misunderstandings to develop.

Multiple Evidence-Based Practices

Many evidence-based practices can fit together because they overlap, interlock, and reinforce one another. Providing just one practice in isolation is, in fact, difficult because the practices are so completely interdependent. Consider this example. Clinicians and administrators sometimes believe that they can implement integrated treatment for co-occurring disorders by training several clinicians to offer addiction counseling, perhaps by having the clinicians use some combination of motivational interviewing and cognitive-behavioral interventions. This approach, however, is incomplete and usually ineffective because people need positive replacements and other supports in order to give up alcohol and drugs. People have great difficulty attaining abstinence unless they can see that their lives will be more satisfying and manageable without substances. Thus, clinicians also need to provide community-integration interventions for their clients. They should help people join Twelve Step groups. Alcoholics Anonymous and other support groups provide role models, new friends, hope, and other supports. Clinicians also need to help their clients find constructive roles. Employment offers a more rewarding long-term role than addiction, but people may need supported employment services to find and succeed in a meaningful job. Clinicians need to use a number of these core clinical skills and evidence-based practices to provide effective treatment.

Stakeholder Perspectives

As clinicians refine their basic skills, their work can help in implementing a specific evidence-based practice. But the key word here is "help" because much of the work of implementing an evidence-based practice needs to be performed by administrators and clinical leaders. As explained in chapter 1, the central tasks of implementation involve preparing, implementing, and maintaining the infrastructure for a specific practice.

Consider the example of supported employment. To implement an evidence-based supported employment program, administrators must determine how to pay for the program, create positions and job descriptions, prepare guidelines for records and billing, hire specific staff members who will supervise and provide employment services, and monitor quality and outcomes. These tasks involve significant preparation of infrastructure, re-engineering of service delivery, and the creation of mechanisms to maintain the services. Professionals with basic skills can easily fill positions offering evidence-based care if the structures supporting the practices are in place.

Clinicians want to be effective and want to enhance their clinical skills, but they are often given negative messages about their clinical work and told that they must adopt an entirely new practice, resulting in resistance as a natural response to such a message. A different message, including positive feedback regarding effectiveness followed by time for extra training to become even more effective, may be more helpful.

Clinical leaders are often reluctant to add evidence-based practices, especially more than one at a time, because they are unfamiliar with the practices themselves and think that they have neither the skills to teach and supervise nor the time to learn. But their concerns suggest another way of proceeding: train clinical leaders and supervisors first, train them on specific skills rather than on complete practices, and help them to become more effective supervisors. Clinical leaders are usually experienced clinicians who carry the clinical culture of a program for years. Investing in their skills is essential and efficient.

They will rapidly acquire new skills, such as motivational interviewing or cognitive-behavioral interventions, and they will help several generations of frontline clinicians learn the skills and apply them appropriately. Their experience will allow them to understand that specific skills underlie multiple evidence-based practices.

Agency and program leaders must protect their agencies, their clinical teams, and themselves. Their organizations must be financially viable, demonstrate effective processes and good outcomes, update infrastructure, satisfy clients and their communities, and retain excellent clinicians. These leaders want to improve care but often are reluctant to create stress in their organizations by announcing that they are going to implement several new evidence-based practices. At the same time, leaders usually recognize that clinicians need to improve their skills continuously and that a core set of skills can inform several evidence-based practices. They also recognize that structural changes may need to occur prior to implementing such practices and that time is needed to make these structural changes as well as to build clinical skills. For example, a mental health agency may not have all the elements of evidence-based integrated treatment. They may not provide addiction treatment, may not be organized in multidisciplinary teams, may not be closely linked with primary health care providers, or may not track key outcomes in their electronic medical records. While clinical leaders are acquiring core skills, agency leaders need time to attend to these types of structural elements.

Administrative leaders at the county, regional, or state level are responsible for several critical tasks. Their commitments encompass client-centered and recovery-oriented care, evidence-based practices, aligning regulations and funding with practices, and continuous training. Addressing these goals simultaneously involves articulating a vision and putting in motion a process of system improvement. The usual approach is to announce and require clinical changes without instituting a process to enable transition. More successful entities first establish training centers that emphasize one or more evidence-based practices by providing training seminars, technical assistance, and, sometimes, learning collaboratives. This approach can encounter difficulties when implementing multiple practices simultaneously. An emphasis on training supervisors in basic skills and how they can be used to construct multiple evidence-based practices may circumvent problems. While initial training is occurring, administrators need to fulfill their responsibilities to ensure that system infrastructure is in place to support implementation and maintenance.

Summary

In this chapter, we have described how multiple evidence-based practices can be implemented by starting with a plan to enhance four basic skills: motivational interviewing, psychoeducation, cognitive-behavioral interventions, and community-integration interventions. This approach emphasizes supporting clinical leaders rather than just the frontline clinicians. Team leaders and supervisors will help many clinicians to develop their skills over time. Basic skills can easily coalesce into a specific evidence-based practice once the infrastructure to support the practice is in place. Clinicians on multidisciplinary teams will gravitate toward specialty roles, but they must all be developing basic skills, and the supports to sustain the practice must be in place, as described in previous chapters.

5

Conclusion

AS STATED IN THE introduction, it takes, according to reviews of the medical literature, about seventeen years for 14 percent of health care research to be implemented and directly impact the public's health (Balas and Boren 2000; Green et al. 2009). If one considers the billions of dollars spent to support biomedical research in the United States and internationally, this would not be categorized as a good "return on investment." This sad state of the science-to-service gap is not lost on anyone. In particular, it has sparked considerable interest in a new area of research called implementation science.

The gap between research and application is also recognized by practitioners in the field. Recently, a group of technical assistance center and treatment professionals were participating in a learning community organized to implement integrated services for co-occurring disorders. The technical assistance center staff were pushing the need for training, which is, as it turns out, what a technical assistance center knows how to do and what it is paid to do. An agency provider spoke up at the meeting and said, "I used to believe our clinicians needed training. So we gave them training, then more training, and then even more training. We probably spent hundreds of thousands of dollars and countless hours of lost productivity in training sessions and workshops. But to be honest, I am not sure it had any real impact on the actual practice in my clinics. The return on investment was horrible." This provider went on to say, "We don't need any more training in practices. We need training in how to implement and sustain practices."

We couldn't agree more.

We have designed this book for the people implementing or trying to implement evidence-based behavioral health practices. We have tried to avoid introducing burdensome research terminology; nevertheless, the findings of implementation science serve as a steady undercurrent to this book. In trying to offer practical advice in the most direct way possible, we have omitted certain details that researchers and implementation scientists may see as essential. To these individuals, we apologize. But for our intended readers, the clinicians and administrators working in the field, we hope this book meets their needs.

Like other "new" fields, implementation science has been around for a while but perhaps been called by other names. Innovative thinking on implementation science is often associated with Everett Rogers, a specialist in rural sociology who described agricultural implementations. More recently, the National Institutes of Health have organized dissemination and implementation (D&I) conferences, and a new journal, *Implementation Science,* has emerged on the topic.

Implementation research is best defined as the scientific study of processes and factors that are associated with successful integration of evidence-based interventions within a particular setting. Although terms such as "technology transfer," "knowledge diffusion," "science-to-service," and many others have been used to describe similar processes, implementation science is an emerging field. Seminal contributions by Rogers (2003) and others catalyzed the early attempts to understand implementation processes. Since then, an abundance of theoretical and conceptual models have been advanced to delineate potentially important processes and factors. The types of interventions being implemented range from agricultural techniques to surgical procedures, and the settings considered include everything from schools to hospitals.

Over the past decade, implementation researchers have devised conceptual models specific to health care. As with the developmental process of any scientific discipline, the early stages have been characterized by theory and model building, with little systematic or confirmatory data and a lack of clear terminology. Different theoretical frameworks and models have generated findings that are not easily compared or contrasted, let alone integrated. A need remains for common measures of implementation strategies and outcomes and for a more systematic way of understanding the factors associated with successful or failed implementations.

> Over the past five years, research on the implementation of behavioral health treatments has been steadily advancing.

Over the past five years, however, research on the implementation of behavioral health treatments has been steadily advancing. Applications of implementation models or frameworks for addressing implementation problems are accumulating, and the terminology is crystallizing. There is also much to be learned from the experience of the early implementation scientists, especially in extending existing work and avoiding previous failures.

Researchers do know that many factors can make or break an implementation. The qualities of the practice and perceptions of it, the larger context (state, region, community, network) within which the treatment organization exists, the characteristics of the organization itself, and, finally, the frontline providers who are expected to deliver the practice—all have their influence.

Interestingly, implementation science embraces the importance of "participatory" research; that is, it recognizes the importance of incorporating the perspectives of all involved at all stages of the practice's development through evaluation to implementation in routine practice. There should be a balance of "push" from those wanting to implement a practice and "pull" from those charged with carrying it out. We have tried to capture all these possible perspectives in this book along with the insights gained from advances in implementation science.

Much of the study of implementation has tended to focus on the implementation of a single practice or innovation, moving from the developers to the frontline providers. The reality is that most treatment providers want to implement a range of practices. Furthermore, treatment providers and systems seek to create an implementation infrastructure so that their agencies don't need to be rebuilt or new staff hired for each new evidence-based practice created. In chapter 4, with these concerns in mind, we described a process for laying a foundation for EBP implementation. Essential skills—including motivational interviewing, cognitive-behavioral therapy, client education, and community-integration interventions—can serve as the core building blocks on which all psychosocial evidence-based practices can be framed. In practice, we have found this approach useful, as have the clinic leaders who have shared their stories with us. In behavioral health research, there has been a surge of interest in identifying core practices or common elements across "name-brand" practices. The early findings are strikingly similar to what we have found in using the four clinical practices as building blocks, as we described in chapter 4.

Over the past three decades, we have worked to develop and test interventions that community treatment providers can use in their everyday practice. Many of these interventions have been proven effective, and some have been widely adopted. This book summarizes what we have learned from the community treatment providers with whom we have partnered. We have highlighted and incorporated the experiences of those providers who have been successful over time in offering their clients evidence-based, proven-effective treatments. In this book, we have also tried to distill much of what can be gleaned from the research, integrate these insights with our practical experience, and communicate them to you in a plain and useful way. We hope that you find this information useful and that it helps you extend your mission to improve the chances for recovery and productive lives among persons with mental illnesses and addictive disorders.

■ ■ ■

Frequently Asked Questions

■ ■ ■

WHEN CONSULTING WITH agencies on evidence-based practices, we are often asked, "What practice should our agency start with?" "What should be the priority practice?" or "How much training is necessary to achieve fidelity?" Although we have experience with each of these questions, we know that there is no cookbook-like formula or perfect strategy for successful implementation. Each agency has to assess its own needs and capacities. In short, one must decide that the evidence-based practice is doable for staff and clearly beneficial to clients to be worth all the effort involved.

The process of implementing a new practice often starts with an agency director or clinical director or perhaps a clinician-leader who has been exposed to an evidence-based practice. This individual assesses the fit of the practice with the agency philosophy or mission. He or she may also consider the complexity of the practice, and perhaps determines if it is realistic for the personnel in the agency to try to implement. Hopefully, the agency also evaluates the evidence for the effectiveness of the practice. Has the practice been scientifically demonstrated to improve treatment outcomes and the prospects for recovery among clients similar to the ones the agency serves? Is this evidence convincing so that the practice is not a "hard sell"? Finally, are clients and families as consumers of services asking for the practice?

What about cost? How much will it cost to learn how to do the practice? This may involve training, time away from revenue-generating activities, the purchase of manuals or workbooks, and support for ongoing trainings or clinical supervision. What will be the return on this investment? Is it clear that the agency's efforts and investments will be outweighed by significant benefits?

As described in chapter 1, it is precisely these questions that should be asked and processed during the preparation or pre-implementation phase. The following questions about the implementation of evidence-based practices in routine behavioral health care settings are, in our experience, common concerns and often raised. We'd like to share our thoughts on these questions here.

How long will start-up take?

Often agency directors consider initial start-up to be time needed for training: "How long will it take my staff to get trained in the intervention?" However, as we have argued, training may be necessary, but training alone is not sufficient to successfully implement an evidence-based practice. Start-up should be conceptualized as a process that includes preparation, training, and then systematic and guided implementation of the practice through supervision and quality, or fidelity, monitoring. Preparation includes the assessment of staff readiness and interest in the practice, as well as consideration of its impact on workflow, time to be allocated to the practice and its implementation, and staff responsibilities.

The length of time for this process varies but should be considered within a timetable of months—not days, weeks, or years. Building up to the training itself—the preparation stage—may take as little as one month or as many as six months. As a rule of thumb, however, start-up generally takes six months.

When should we hold the first training?

Begin training at the end of the preparation stage or early in the implementation stage. This is generally after agency attitudes, readiness, workflow, and other contingencies have been considered and the costs and rewards of the practice have been carefully reviewed with decision makers and implementers. In addition, the first training should take place when the leaders sponsoring the training are convinced of the effectiveness of the practice, the feasibility of implementing it, the capacity of the staff to carry it out, and its overall fit with agency mission. The training should not be conceptualized as the point when the staff members are "won over" to the practice or as an end point to the start-up. It is the culmination of the process of implementation and the launch of a "hands-on" implementation process.

Our state/agency has a policy that contradicts one of the fidelity items. Should we follow the agency/state policy and follow only the other fidelity items?

As an initial response, we would ask for verification that the state policy, in fact, contradicts a fidelity item. Such verification should be made verbally with state agency officials, as well as by examining the line(s) ostensibly stating the conflicting policy. In our experience, these supposed contradictions are often myths. When one searches for evidence of the policy conflict, it cannot be found.

If a state or agency policy presents a barrier to carrying out a practice with fidelity (for example, it bars offering housing to a person who has not achieved stable abstinence), then we encourage you to challenge the policy with the evidence for the practice. Should the implementation of the practice be delayed because of a single policy barrier when all others are feasible? No.

We agree with most of the principles of the evidence-based practice we are implementing, but we think we have a better way of doing one of the principles. Is it okay?

In light of local customs, cultural and gender-specific concerns, and other factors, implementers often want to modify an evidence-based practice to make it better fit an agency's needs or clients. Most evidence-based practices have been tested under a variety of conditions with a range of clients and with a heterogeneous group of behavioral health disorders. At the preparatory stage of implementation, reviewers should consider these issues when evaluating the evidence for the effectiveness of a practice. That being said, it may be that some adaptation is necessary to improve the fit of the practice with your realities. Caution is needed, however, whenever changing a practice. Evidence-based practices have been studied and found to be effective when delivered competently and as designed. It is quite possible that in modifying a practice, it will be fundamentally changed and in the process may lose some important ingredients to its effectiveness. To minimize the number and extent of these adaptations, it is a good idea to refer to a fidelity scale and consult with a technical assistance center expert. Also, when possible, discuss the change with the developers of the practice. They should be able to describe what the "core" components of the evidence-based practice are versus those that may be modified.

We agree with most of the principles of the evidence-based practice we are implementing, but implementing one of the principles is too expensive. Is it okay to skip this one?

Before dropping a component of the practice, you should consider that in subtracting it, you could end up removing a key element in the practice's effectiveness. To avoid making this untimely discovery only after you have already invested in implementation, it is critical to evaluate a practice at the outset, at the preparatory stage. This effort can save time and costs and avoid faulty implementation of practices.

For example, you may have decided to implement IDDT. If you carefully review IDDT early on, you'll recognize that IDDT involves stage-wise treatment and assertive outreach to clients during engagement. If your clinical staff are solely office-based and you do not have case management staff for outreach or community-integration activities, then IDDT is probably not the best option for you to implement. It is better to recognize what your agency has the capacity to tackle than alter major principles or components of a practice.

Should we implement all the evidence-based practices at once, or should we spread implementation out over time? If we stagger start-up, which evidence-based practice should we start with?

As described in chapter 4, there are four foundational skills for practitioners in behavioral health care: motivational interviewing, cognitive-behavioral therapy, psychoeducation, and community-integration. These four core skills are the building blocks of specific evidence-based practices, such as *Integrating Combined Therapies* (a curriculum in Hazelden's Co-occurring Disorders Program), IMR, and IDDT.

Motivational interviewing is an essential skill for client assessment and in the early phases of treatment. Client education can be integrated with most motivational interviewing approaches, for instance in developing the discrepancy between clients' understanding of their current functioning and how they would like to be. Cognitive-behavioral therapy comes into play when a person is in the active change process and later in the recovery maintenance stage—after initial changes have already been made. Community-integration skills are used when engaging persons not consistently accessing services and with clients in the recovery maintenance stage. For example, these skills are an important part of supported employment and Twelve Step facilitation approaches.

Assuming clinicians are new or require ongoing in-service training, building evidence-based practices on these four skills would be an excellent strategy. Of these four skills, one might start with training in motivational interviewing and community-integration approaches and then move to mastering cognitive-behavioral therapy and client education.

How quickly should we enroll clients?

After training is completed and access to expert technical assistance and continued clinical supervision and/or quality monitoring is in place, client enrollment should begin immediately. It is only by applying the new skills, receiving feedback and encouragement, and refining these skills in actual practice that effective implementation will take place.

Should we collect outcome data?

In behavioral health care, practitioners can record many outcomes and dimensions of outcomes. Some outcomes are measures made "within treatment," such as those noting baseline functioning and the appropriate, guideline-based assignment of treatments or levels of care. Other within-treatment outcomes may be "process" measures. One can measure program access (for example, by recording those clients showing up for an initial service) or engagement (by recording those continuing in services once initiated) and retention (by noting how many completed a "full course" of a time-limited service). Finally, providers can gather "during-treatment" outcomes. These include outcomes related to symptom change or even satisfaction with services. Assessing these factors while a person is still in active treatment enables the provider to adjust the treatment plan in the event client progress is not positive or to continue with the treatment plan if its benefits have been observed and measured.

These during-treatment measures are actually very useful to the ongoing clinical process, program evaluation, and quality-assurance efforts, and they can be used to document the benefit of an EBP implementation. As "dashboard indicators," these measures should be collected and, to the extent possible, relayed to key parties (clinician, client, program director) in real time. Most agencies do not necessarily have the capacity to gather outcomes in real time, so they try to collect these data on a weekly, monthly, or quarterly basis.

Traditional outcome data include data on clients' functioning post-treatment (after treatment has ended). Sometimes, these types of outcomes are gathered at three months, six months, or up to one year after a treatment episode has ended. These types of outcomes are difficult for many agencies to collect because clients are often lost to follow-up. And clients who have relocated or who are dissatisfied do not respond to survey requests. Furthermore, if one truly believes that mental health and substance use disorders are chronic conditions that require ongoing management, outcomes taken post-treatment may be an unfair test of treatment effectiveness. No one would try to assess hypertension three, six, or twelve months after high blood pressure medications have been discontinued and then judge the efficacy of the medication based on these follow-ups. So, too, may be the case with behavioral health evaluations.

If post-treatment follow-up data are gathered, it is important to consider the cost of collecting reliable and valid outcome information, the representativeness of the data sample, and the accuracy of reports relying on self-reported data alone. Nevertheless, quarterly to annual reporting of these outcome data may provide the program with some means to evaluate its services.

How should we select a technical assistance center?

A technical assistance center should have clear expertise in the four core skills and the evidence-based practices being implemented, and it should have facility in working within mental health and addiction (that is, integrated) treatment contexts. In evaluating a technical assistance center, an agency must be confident in the center's experience with implementation (not just training), including its ability to provide ongoing supervision and fidelity monitoring and to facilitate a learning community.

How often do we need to conduct a fidelity assessment?

When a practice like IDDT, supported employment, or IMR is being established during the implementation stage, it is best to conduct fidelity assessments often. This may involve carrying out fidelity assessments at six-month intervals or even quarterly. In monitoring individual or group therapies (such as motivational interviewing, motivational enhancement therapy, or cognitive-behavioral therapy), an agency should conduct adherence and competence assessments on at least 25 percent of all sessions until acceptable implementation has occurred. These assessments can be carried out via direct observation or audio/video tape review.

Once services-related fidelity has been achieved, annual assessments are appropriate, unless a change in key staffing or programming has occurred. These events may precipitate a fidelity check.

It is appropriate to observe therapy adherence and competence on a monthly or quarterly basis. To sustain clinical practices, these strategies can then be used in clinical supervision and staff development.

Who should conduct fidelity assessments? Can sites self-assess?

We appreciate the pull to conduct one's own fidelity assessment—it can save time, money, and perhaps avoid the anxiety associated with having an outsider's evaluation. However, a number of studies have shown that these self-assessments tend to be inflated and therefore invalid. It's better to have outside evaluators conduct fidelity assessments.

But is a self-assessment better than no fidelity assessment? Yes, but as a screening tool, not an official review of capability. Self-assessments are best used to prepare for an upcoming independent fidelity assessment.

Fidelity assessments should be conducted by persons affiliated with the technical assistance center, the state agency, or academic research groups with experience in conducting the fidelity check in question. Evidence-based practices are not all alike, so it is imperative that the assessment be performed by a person or team with specific expertise in the fidelity scale being used.

Once we've collected the fidelity data, what do we do with it?

Fidelity scale data are best used to support the hard work of the clinical staff and team members who have dedicated their efforts to implementing the practice. They are measures of an implementation's success. Fidelity scale data can also be used to examine variations across groups implementing the same practice. These data can be used to guide and measure quality improvement. Lastly, if your agency is a member of a learning community, fidelity scale information can help you communicate with other community members about barriers to and elements of successful implementation.

Are fidelity assessors certified?

There is no formal process for certifying fidelity assessors. As regulatory and funding agencies mandate that evidence-based practices be provided, this may change.

At present, the qualifications that fidelity assessors need can be obtained from your state behavioral health agency or the developers of the intervention or by contacting the Dartmouth Psychiatric Research Center.

How many fidelity assessors are needed to conduct an assessment?

We recommend that there be two members to a fidelity assessment team.

How do we decide if our fidelity assessment score is good enough?

All fidelity measures have a cutoff score for "acceptable" delivery of a practice or service. In some cases, regulatory agencies may set the standard for programs they fund or for certain levels of care. In one state, all intensive outpatient programs are required to be operating at the Dual Diagnosis Capable (DDC) level on the Dual Diagnosis Capability in Addiction Treatment (DDCAT) Index. This is not the highest rating on the DDCAT, but it indicates that the agency has the clinical practices, policies, and workforce expertise that enable delivery of the basics of integrated care.

At the pre-implementation stage, you can target specific fidelity-scale criteria and establish a timeline for achieving them. Your progress in meeting these criteria can serve as a formal charting of your course to successful implementation.

Interview with an Agency Director

THE FOLLOWING INTERVIEW represents the story of an individual agency and its efforts to implement evidence-based practices. The Hazelden editor spoke to the agency leader, hoping to get some insight into practitioners' real-world experience in implementing a complex practice. What worked? What were the challenges? What would the agency recommend? This account is not intended to serve as a template for all practitioners. However, within this account, several common themes emerge: the place of training, the role of agency leaders and clinical supervisors, the challenges and strategies for implementing practices, and the incentives and sources of support for agency change.

We include the following interview as a case example and hope that it will provide some insights and strategies for our readers.

* * *

Buddy Garfinkle is the associate executive director at Bridgeway, a mental health rehabilitation services provider based in Elizabeth, New Jersey. Our editor spoke with him about the agency's experiences in implementing evidence-based practices in behavioral health.

Can you tell me about your agency and the clients you serve?

We work with people with severe and persistent mental illness. In most of our programs, it has to be one of the major axis-I diagnoses: schizophrenia, major depression, bipolar disorder, schizoaffective disorder, and delusional disorders. We're not working with people who have neuroses or adjustment disorders. Our service population has been carrying these diagnoses for a long time.

Ours is a very high-intensity service. You could call us a niche provider because this is the 5 percent that uses 50 percent of the resources in behavioral health and physical health. Ours is a very high-need population.

What's your background? How did you start at the agency?

I started work in New York City doing outreach to the homeless and housing development [residents] back in the late '80s, early '90s. My first real work with our population was in setting up community residences, which we called at the time MICA-residences, in New York. And when assertive community treatment—which we call PACT in New Jersey—was established, my present boss was looking for a director and I happened to meet him by chance and he hired me in 1996. [PACT is Program for Assertive Community Treatment.]

So for a number of years, PACT was my world, and in that time, we've grown from three PACT teams to nine PACT teams, and we also run the Training and Technical Assistance Center for PACT in New Jersey. We train all the new teams and staff for the thirty-one PACT teams in New Jersey. So that's what I've been doing.

In around 2002, 2003, when assertive community treatment [ACT] came to New York, the Office of Mental Health in New York was looking for a training entity to train their new teams, and because we already had a training institute set up, our agency became the trainers for implementation of ACT. I believe they [the Office of Mental Health] were training fifty-two teams all at once, and paralleled the beginning of the evidence-based practice story for Bridgeway. As New York State was moving into the assertive community treatment–service delivery system, they also wanted to make sure that the teams were going to be evidence-based practice teams.

How did you begin adding evidence-based practices to your services?

While I was teaching ACT, [trainers from Dartmouth and IMR developer Susan Gingerich] were teaching some of the other evidenced-based practices, and we did some coordination. I asked Susan if I could attend the IMR trainings, and of course she said yes. And while I saw where [implementing ACT and IMR simultaneously as new practices] wasn't going to work for New York initially, I saw how IMR was going to work for us in New Jersey, because we already had our ACT teams set up, and we saw ACT as the perfect platform on which to layer IMR as an evidence-based practice.

So your agency settled on implementing IMR?

We were thinking: should we do IMR? Or start with IDDT [integrated dual disorders treatment]? We knew about IDDT because select Bridgeway staff were invited to those trainings as well. But we thought—as a psych rehab agency working within the recovery model—that recovery from mental illness pertained to everybody, whereas IDDT did not.

How did you begin implementing IMR?

I could see how the teams that I was working with in ACT were struggling with implementing IMR. At Bridgeway we discussed it with our core management team, our clinical staff managers, and said that we need to be methodical and calculate how we could make this practice work and not just use it for ACT but really use it for all of our programs. The agency has a number of different programs: day treatment (which we call partial care), supportive housing, a PATH program for homeless outreach, and a pretty well-developed ACT program. In thinking about our options with some of my peers and in seeing how IMR is set up, we realized that we didn't have an even playing field in terms of the staff's clinical core competencies, or the counseling skills that you need to have in place to do IMR well.

We agreed to implement IMR, but in order to develop the staff's clinical skills, we decided that we were going to hire a motivational interviewing [MI] expert, a local Ph.D. professor. Training was to be for a small group; we weren't going to teach everybody initially. It was [for] a group of twenty people. He [the trainer] taught us motivational interviewing in a classroom model with homework.

How did you identify the small group to be trained in motivational interviewing? What role were they [the group] going to play at the agency?

Our clinical supervisors and the people who had at least a modicum of training in motivational interviewing were included in the group. They were going to be our internal champions. That was key. So anybody who had had some training in MI.

And at that time, similar to now, if you asked practitioners in a room "How many people have been trained in MI?" 65 percent of the hands would go up. And if you would say, "Okay, how many of you would be willing to show me how to do it?" you might get 10 percent. Many staff members have been to classroom training, but they haven't practiced the MI skills. They haven't sufficiently learned it [MI]; it hasn't been supported within their agencies. We were determined to not let that happen.

We had twenty people who were trained in MI.

So all the focus was on IMR and motivational interviewing as a building block for IMR?

Yes. At the same time, we were invited to New York ACT trainings in IDDT. We attended six trainings, and we saw how motivational interviewing and CBT [cognitive-behavioral therapy] were the foundational skills in IDDT, reinforcing our original thought that we really needed to have these skills established before we could launch any of the other evidence-based practices.

Okay. So, in specific, how did you organize the initial training in MI for the agency leaders' group?

Between the MI training that we had from our expert in New Jersey and the IDDT trainings that we had attended in New York, we developed training for our staff. And we just borrowed, mixed and matched; we didn't create anything particularly new, but we saw what was going to apply for us.

What we did—before we rolled any of it out to the rest of the agency—was set up two regional groups with co-facilitators. I ran one group. Another director had responsibility for the other group, each with a co-facilitator. We reinforced and worked on MI, breaking it down into each skill, first the OARS, the micro-skills, and then the eliciting-change talk as they pertain to the stages of change. [OARS are the motivational interviewing skills of open-ended questions, affirmations, reflective listening, and summaries. The stages of change are precontemplation, contemplation, preparation, action, and maintenance.]

We were meeting about every two or three weeks. After MI sessions, you [the participants in the training] reported back to the training group, having completed a skills checklist demonstrating which MI skills you were using in sessions while providing the rationale for choosing the skill to the group. And while it wasn't direct observation, it was pretty strong in terms of the feedback that people were getting. We wanted these twenty people to be the real champions of this endeavor.

How did you bring the training in motivational interviewing to all the staff?

We had representation of all of our clinical teams within the work groups, and after about four months, we rolled out an agency-wide training on motivational interviewing. All clinical staff were involved. For clinical staff who thought it didn't even pertain to them, we said, "Tough luck." Our belief was that these implementations were going to flow into a vacuum if we didn't train everyone agency-wide. We believed that an agency-wide training would support the culture shift necessary for establishing best practices throughout the agency.

Often in multidisciplinary or interdisciplinary teams, people will attend training, and then they'll come back to the team and they'll get a nice pat on the back and a "Good for you, kid. That's great. I hope you get to use it." Staff may be excited about what they've learned, but it's not supported because no one on the team has been trained in the same content. Having seen how good training can go for naught, we decided ours was going to be an agency-wide initiative.

We rolled out MI, using the same training model: all staff on the clinical teams on all of our teams were to be trained. So at the time, it must have been [that] about

150 people were asked to work with a person served who was in the contemplation stage using the MI skills and then to come back to the team to describe their sessions. In the weekly clinical meetings, [trainees] had to present what they had done through the MI lens with the persons served. So it was very focused on just working within those skills.

So was the original group's training in MI complete at this point? What was this group's role in the agency-wide training?

Those regional groups did not stop meeting. The staff who had gotten the original training needed to be supported as the clinical champions to reinforce the practice.

The original group of twenty was getting the extra training and supervision within the smaller groups. They would discuss supervision issues that they were having. We wanted that original group to be steps ahead of everybody else, because they were going to have to help staff to develop their skills. If so, we wanted to give that extra bumped-up support to this group.

Meanwhile, we were learning only MI. We were not doing IMR yet. We were not doing IDDT. We were just focusing on developing motivational interviewing skills.

And how did the agency-wide training in MI go?

We added that [training in MI] to the orientation for all new staff. So I guess this went on for about six months, just MI. We wanted it to be embedded in our agency culture, so we took our time with it.

As in any kind of initiative where you have 150 people or so [participating], you're going to have different levels of expertise. But staff were certainly excited about it, and even for those people who couldn't demonstrate the skills that well, they could certainly speak to it. And, you know, that was pretty good. We changed some of our documentation forms to show the skills that we were trying to implement in our agency.

Did you see any changes in staff practices?

MI was like a gift to us, because when people served are contemplating change, they are ambivalent. Staff would say things like, "Oh . . . here we go again. What am I going to do with this person? They're not ready [to make changes]." And now we had specific skills to help staff make choices, direct the session, and attend to their readiness, so it really felt like a gift. And this was not just for bachelor's-level staff, but it was master's-level staff who hadn't yet developed an enhanced level of clinical expertise. . . .

An issue within a community-based agency is that there's nothing static about staffing. You may have practitioners that come and go. You have new people coming in at a fairly steady rate. We didn't have excessive turnover at the time, because what we were creating was a practicing and learning environment. In spite of the relatively low salaries, staff felt that they were part of a changing agency culture, which was pretty cool. When you're creating a learning culture within an agency that is a practicing agency, you start to see the retention levels go up. And that was by design as well, because we wanted to create this environment where we felt that even if people were going to eventually move on we were going to give them skills and knowledge to take off into their future. The learning environment was one of the ways of keeping staff in the agency.

In working with your consumers, did you see any special benefits of using MI?
MI gave us a skill set to connect with people in a way that wasn't necessarily goal-focused. We were working with people who had been in and out of the system. Plus our PACT programs throughout the state, like the original ACT model, really are for people who had multiple hospitalizations and were often mistrustful of providers.

We had lots of people who were in early stages [of change], and not real goal-focused but questioning, "Well, what are you going to do for me?" And this is even years into the program. So when you are the recipient of people coming out of state hospitals, local hospitals, and the people you see are not stable in terms of their course of illness or their community adaptation, you have to connect with people and build trust. You can't rush into it, so MI was something that we found that worked very, very well throughout our program. People were even using it in the PATH program for homeless outreach.

Once you'd felt people had received training in motivational interviewing, what were the next steps? Did you move to implementing IMR?
When we felt that we had at least a fairly level playing field in terms of people being able to demonstrate the skills, certainly speak to the skills, we then moved into CBT. I developed an agency-wide training with another staff person coming out of our supported employment program who had been trained in CBT.

We developed a CBT training, not nearly as elaborate as the MI training because, for a psychiatric rehabilitation agency, CBT is very much in line with the work that we've been doing. We're pretty good at teaching people skills, because that's what psychiatric rehabilitation is about. So we didn't have to make the training that elaborate. We also didn't pretend to be cognitive-behavioral therapists; we took much more of a skills development orientation.

So we taught people the principles of cognitive restructuring. We taught people concepts such as schema and how to use schema worksheets, without any illusion that people were really going to master it. But we wanted to focus mostly on the methodologies of teaching skills—like Susan Gingerich in *Building Social Support,* the practice tape that she did for IMR. She does it so artfully and lays out how you model the skills within a role-play. That resonated very, very nicely. So even within the CBT training, I used that module to show people how to set up a role-play, giving feedback, appreciative feedback, constructive feedback—those kinds of skills.

We used the same regional groups to set up the CBT training, we kept the same structure, and we rolled it out to staff, but we didn't need the six months to finish the training. It was more like a two- or three-month implementation, and staff mastered it pretty quickly. We emphasized the stages of change concept, that when people move into the latter stages of change, preparation and particularly action and then maintenance, you [as practitioner] are now moving into your CBT skill set.

Did you find it useful to start with MI and move to CBT, to allow you to focus on the stages of change?

We knew that MI was much more pertinent to those earlier stages, and we also knew that MI was going to be very new for some of our people [staff]. Different folks within the agency had some training. We had one or two people who were pretty good at it. And we knew that MI was going to entail much more.

People struggled with MI, as we expected. Staff are ready to jump into solutions, and they felt that there was this pressure from funding sources to get people served into the action stage quickly, because you need to see results and positive outcomes. But people don't change that way. And MI gives you permission to slow that process down, because people aren't ready for change necessarily within our time frames.

Can you talk a little bit about what kind of changes you started to see once your staff had this training in motivational interviewing and CBT?

It all moved right into IMR, an agency-wide implementation of IMR. We taught IMR and we used [the IMR authors Kim Mueser's and Susan Gingerich's] materials and the demonstration tapes. That training wasn't that hard, because once you have those skills [MI and CBT], it really just becomes curriculum and then practice.

So MI and CBT training set up work on the IMR program? How did the implementation of this practice proceed?

The IMR implementation was really wonderful because it further embedded the culture shift in the agency, and it was our first evidence-based practice. (PACT was really our first evidence-based practice, but it is a programmatic structure, not a curriculum requiring clinical skills.)

Once we moved into IMR, with the focus on recovery, staff really felt that we were doing something of importance and that furthered the enthusiasm about the practices that we had learned. In using MI and CBT in conjunction with IMR, we kind of felt like we were using those clinical skills that we worked so hard on. The beauty of IMR is not in its sophistication; it's the opposite. The beauty of it is that it's laid out so nicely, and you don't have to be a master clinician to implement it fairly well.

I also think that with IMR, when we got into some of the latter modules on coping with stress and some of the work with psychotic systems, staff really believed that they were bumping up their clinical interventions and were really proud of their ability to work with persons served, and there was some really good teaching embedded in the practice. And with that, it motivated us to learn more.

At the time, after our original implementation, [IMR developers] Kim Mueser and Susan Gingerich had come to New Jersey to pilot IMR with some agencies, and although we were only partially into the implementation, we joined, and of course it was very, very helpful. They set up a supervision model. We followed the Dartmouth EBP model of phone calls [as consultation], but they also would come to New Jersey and would teach supervision of IMR. And I would have some private discussions with them, because they appreciated that we were working really hard at the IMR implementation. So it was a really nice exchange at the time, and it was a great statewide push in New Jersey to make IMR stick. I think there were like ten agencies that were in this pilot. And with the extra support and the supervision trainings, it was a very big, helpful tool. IMR in New Jersey and particularly here at Bridgeway got a real hold, and with the state very invested in it at the time, I think it was helpful, within Bridgeway, to see that this was a practice that was going to stick as a core practice.

It sounds like you felt that training in MI and CBT was a good groundwork for IMR. How about the IDDT and supported employment programs at your agency?

Through my work with New York and their ACT initiative and exposure to IMR and my talks with Kim and Susan, we figured out pretty early on that MI and CBT were the core competencies for all the evidence-based practices. If you have those skills as part of your agency culture, then the rest of implementation would basically come down to learning and implementing curriculum.

We decided at our agency that IMR was the best place to start and that we would implement one evidenced-based practice at a time. Slow it down. Make sure that people have all their clinical skills before you launch into the practices.

Can you talk a little bit about how you implemented IDDT?

I trained the PACT program managers, the clinical supervisors, the team leaders, and the CADCs [certified alcohol and drug centers] in IDDT over the course of about four months, and we did it classroom training style. We probably had about thirty people in the room. And using the same method, starting off with the screening tools and assessments and all of the instruments that had been tested for reliability, using the curriculum and the toolkit, we moved slowly through the training, and staff really benefited.

Each session lasted three hours, allowing staff to go back to perform their jobs for the rest of the day. They were assigned IDDT homework, and then before each session, I'd choose some people who were to present their homework to the group and then we'd discuss the sessions using a group supervision format. We developed wonderful group cohesion. The team leaders were learning along with their co-occurring specialists, ensuring that it became part of the PACT teams' practice. We have learned the lesson: if leadership isn't involved, then forget it. You're wasting your time.

We had everybody involved, and we had such a positive learning experience with IDDT that the participants didn't want the training to end. So when we got into the latter stages [of change and the interventions used then], particularly CBT, I used a few different dual disorders manuals, where staff could teach the actual skills, things like refusal skills and coping with cravings. We wanted to move fairly quickly through the curriculum, but staff insisted on taking their time, hoping to refine the skills. It was pretty funny, because while they really felt like they were learning, I knew they were stalling. They liked the group cohesion. And I didn't push back because I felt like the more learning that we did, the more it was going to become ingrained in their daily practice. And after about four months I said, "Okay, enough already, use it." But they had already been using the modules since they had homework. After each module, they put the concepts into practice right away, helping them to retain the skills. We used this training model, and IDDT became a very important practice within our PACT program.

Well, we didn't stop there.... I shared the IDDT curriculum with an agency colleague. He trained other programs in the agency. He continues to do advanced MI training, CBT training, and IDDT training throughout the agency.

I was interested in what you said about training in relation to hanging on to staff. Can you talk about that?

You create a certain kind of ideal when staff feel that they are learning skills that they can immediately use. With these implementations, you know, we wanted to create a model of practice and communicate that these clinical skills will help you to get better at your job. So when you're in an environment where people are learning and practicing together, you forge a culture that encompasses learning and practice. You create a spirit where staff enthusiastically report to their peers some of the successes that they've had, and they get really excited about their work.

I can remember this one staff member, a vocational specialist, who had been involved in the original MI training. He was talking to a person served whom he had known for a few years. He was practicing reflective listening skills, and he came back with this look of wonder on his face. He said, "Do you know that he has eight grandchildren?" His team members said, "No, we didn't know that. And we've been working with this guy for years!" Through the practice of reflective listening, this man opened up because our staff person had connected with him in a different way. I mean, that's reinforcement. That reinforces those practices.

That's great to see how training can have an immediate impact. Have you found other ways to reinforce a practice?

The IMR progress note . . . was wonderful for us, because it reinforced on a day-to-day basis the learning . . . the skills used. So I just love that. We modified that progress note to support our own implementation.

So in a sense you're using the progress note to track not only the consumer's progress but also the facilitator's in using the new clinician skills?

That's right. It's not exactly only progress-note oriented. It's more a reinforcement for you, the clinician, to use to remind you of the skills you should be using in your everyday work. On each progress note, we asked staff to write the individual's goal that he or she is working on and the person's stage of change. So if you're talking about [someone in] an earlier stage of change, then you're probably going to be checking off some of the MI skills utilized, which will then be spoken to within the progress note. And then, of course, you describe how the person responded to your intervention.

Can you talk a little bit about sustaining a practice? We've talked a bit about how your agency implemented an evidence-based practice, but what would you say is key to sustaining it?

You sustain it through supervision—individual and group supervision. In your clinical meetings, you're going to ask people, individual practitioners, to present what they did through a certain evidenced-based practice lens. Staff describe an IMR session or an IDDT session.

You also sustain it by developing outcome measures. Some of the outcome measures are our recovery measures for persons served, which is what the funders want to see. But you want separate outcome measures tied to the EBP implementation. So if I have, let's say, a unit of sixty people on a caseload, we're going to set a measure that says 25 percent of the people served within the course of a year are going to be getting IMR services. If you have 25 percent [of consumers participating in IMR], that means each clinician will have provided IMR services to two people served.

We tie the implementation measures to performance appraisals. We have kind of an interesting model with our performance appraisals, and we're pretty religious about this. We don't wait until the end of the year to say, "Okay, how did you do?" But in our weekly or every-other-week supervision, we go through the goals that staff set at the beginning of the year. A major portion of the appraisal is based on recovery-based and EBP implementation outcome measures. And they're quantified. All team members are responsible for working toward these measurable goals.

So if, let's say, 20 percent of the people served who have addiction issues move from pre-contemplation into action, at the end of the year, we're going to be compiling the data. We're going to be measuring movement toward behavior change, and even if I personally didn't have a whole lot to do with an individual's progress and my teammates' success, we all get credit for progress. So we create this kind of *esprit de corps* around some of these outcome measures.

Do you set these benchmarks for many of your programs?

Yes. We establish benchmarks that are connected to the evidenced-based practice. Before we establish targets, we need to create a benchmark. We may establish that 25 percent of the caseload with addiction issues will have a relapse prevention plan. At the end of the year, we are going to be evaluated on that measure. We know that PACT is required to demonstrate low re-hospitalization rates. Since we have historical data covering fifteen years, we have established benchmarks. We're going to say only 10 percent of the caseload are going to be re-hospitalized in a given year. We are then evaluated on this measure as a group.

The agency has developed a strategic plan, and the goals set trickle down to the individual practice. As an agency, we establish that we are a best-practices agency with an emphasis on evidence-based practices. And we're always trying to create that thread between what we're trying to do as an agency [and] the individual practitioner.

And this is part of the effort to sustain these practices at the agency?

We've been fortunate in holding on to the team leaders who have been involved in the EBP trainings. But the other issue in terms of sustainability is that you want to hire from within, because as people get their advanced degrees, they've been part of this learning process and best practices. If somebody comes from the outside, it is challenging because the new leader has to catch up with their supervisees to learn the EBPs. Hiring from within, in terms of maintaining an agency culture, is critical.

So group supervision and outcome measures help in reinforcing these new practices. Are there other changes that take place to accommodate these new practices?

I've talked before about the progress note. All of the forms that we have within the agency have now been developed to support the evidence-based practices. So if you have a recovery plan, within the recovery plan we'll complete [a section called] Developing Goals. You have to write where the person is within their change process toward a certain goal. If the person is in the preparation stage in the development of their recovery plan, their behavioral objectives have to reflect the things that they're going to do to attain their goal. Staff interventions reflect or correspond to what the person is doing. We [practitioners] read these progress notes and plans aloud to each other to support learning.

All goal plans and progress notes have to be read. So let's say a practitioner is reading a goal plan for his or her team. The practitioner is going to be questioned by the team leader or team member on how the intervention corresponds to the person's goals and objectives. . . . We may see that a person served wants to cope with psychotic symptoms, leading us to suggest an IMR module that can help with coping strategies. Staff feel supported, and they feel like they're learning when you make these suggestions. So those of us who are the managers or even provide the clinical oversight have to remind people of the EBP learning. We have to maintain the EBP focus, because staff get caught up in the day-to-day responsibilities, and it's so easy to fall back into just providing those linear, concrete services. And we're not about just doing "the day-to-day stuff." We're about teaching skills and helping people to recover. . . .

So we always have agency initiatives. And another thing about retention—and the way to keep enthusiasm going—is that you don't stop implementations. You don't sit on your laurels. You don't say, "Okay, we've now established ourselves as a best-practices agency." You have to keep the learning moving forward, and I think staff then feel like they're part of something special.

Appendix

Implementation Resources

Implementing Evidence-Based Practices: An Agency's Tasks

Prioritization

Implementation Dimension	Definition
Attitude	Clinic leaders offer expressions of support for the implementation of the evidence-based practice
Understanding	Understanding of the evidence-based practice is present or being sought
Mandate	The mental health authority requires that this evidence-based practice be offered
Money	Financial backing for the implementation of this evidence-based practice is available

Leadership

Implementation Dimension	Definition
Responsibility	A program leader has the responsibility and authority to implement this evidence-based practice
Leadership Skills	Leadership skills for implementation and delivery of the evidence-based practice are present
Plan Enactment	A plan is in place for the implementation of the evidence-based practice
Engagement	Efforts are being made to build active support among other stakeholders for offering this evidence-based practice
Plan Sustaining	There is a plan for the sustained offering of this evidence-based practice
Change Culture	The agency culture is open to the changes needed to implement this evidence-based practice

Workforce

Implementation Dimension	Definition
Staffing	Attempts are being made to meet the staffing requirements of the evidence-based practice
Personnel Action	Personnel problems that detract from implementation and delivery of the evidence-based practice are addressed
Skill Mastery	The skills needed by practitioners to offer the evidence-based practice are present or being sought
Training	Training in the evidence-based practice is being offered
Supervision	Clinical supervision of the evidence-based practice is being offered

Workflow

Implementation Dimension	Definition
Staff Meetings	A meeting structure that supports the evidence-based practice is present
Documentation	Documentation practices support the evidence-based practice
Support Staff	Support staff function to support the evidence-based practice
Physical Environment	The physical environment supports the implementation of the evidence-based practice
Policies	Policies supporting the evidence-based practice are present

Reinforcement

Implementation Dimension	Definition
Penetration	Measures of program penetration are collected and used to improve the evidence-based practice
Outcome Monitoring	Client outcomes are collected and monitored in order to improve the evidence-based practice
Fidelity	Measures of fidelity are collected and used to improve the evidence-based practice
Rewards	Success is celebrated in order to reinforce the evidence-based practice
Credentialing	Programs are credentialed to reinforce the evidence-based practice
Feedback	Feedback from practitioners and clients is solicited and used to monitor and improve the evidence-based practice

Supported Employment Fidelity Scale

(Content Revised in 2008)

Rater: _____ Date: _____

Site: _____

Note: Fidelity reviewers fill out this scale using the notes they took while visiting the organization.

Data sources:

MIS	Management Information System
DOC	Document review: clinical records, agency policy and procedures
INT	Interviews with clients, employment specialists, mental health staff, VR counselors, families, employers
OBS	Observation (e.g., team meeting, shadowing employment specialists)
ISP	Individualized Service Plan

Directions: Circle one anchor number for each criterion.

Item Score: _____

STAFFING

Criterion **1**

Caseload size: Employment specialists have individual employment caseloads. The maximum caseload for any full-time employment specialist is 20 or fewer clients.

DATA SOURCE		ANCHOR
MIS, DOC, INT	1	Ratio of 41 or more clients per employment specialist
	2	Ratio of 31–40 clients per employment specialist
	3	Ratio of 26–30 clients per employment specialist
	4	Ratio of 21–25 clients per employment specialist
	5	Ratio of 20 or fewer clients per employment specialist

Directions: Circle one anchor number for each criterion.

Item Score:_____

STAFFING

Criterion 2

Employment services staff: Employment specialists provide only employment services.

DATA SOURCE		ANCHOR
MIS, DOC, INT	1	Employment specialists provide employment services less than 60% of the time.
	2	Employment specialists provide employment services 60–74% of the time.
	3	Employment specialists provide employment services 75–89% of the time.
	4	Employment specialists provide employment services 90–95% of the time.
	5	Employment specialists provide employment services 96% or more of the time.

Directions: Circle one anchor number for each criterion.

Item Score:_____

STAFFING

Criterion 3

Vocational generalists: Each employment specialist carries out all phases of employment service, including intake, engagement, assessment, job placement, job coaching, and follow-along supports before step down to less intensive employment support from another MH practitioner. (Note: It is not expected that each employment specialist will provide benefits counseling to his or her clients. Referrals to a highly trained benefits counselor are in keeping with high fidelity; see item #1 in "Services.")

DATA SOURCE		ANCHOR
MIS, DOC, INT, OBS	1	Employment specialist only provides vocational referral service to vendors and other programs.
	2	Employment specialist maintains caseload but refers clients to other programs for vocational services.
	3	Employment specialist provides one to four phases of the employment service (e.g., intake, engagement, assessment, job development, job placement, job coaching, and follow-along supports).
	4	Employment specialist provides five phases of employment service but not the entire service.
	5	Employment specialist carries out all six phases of employment service (i.e., program intake, engagement, assessment, job development/job placement, job coaching, and follow-along supports).

Directions: Circle one anchor number for each criterion.

Item Score:_____

ORGANIZATION

Criterion **1**

Integration of rehabilitation with mental health treatment through team assignment: Employment specialists are part of up to two mental health treatment teams from which at least 90% of the employment specialist's caseload is comprised.

DATA SOURCE		ANCHOR
MIS, DOC, INT, OBS	1	Employment specialists are part of a vocational program that functions separately from the mental health treatment.
	2	Employment specialists are attached to three or more mental health treatment teams. **OR** Clients are served by individual mental health practitioners who are not organized into teams. **OR** Employment specialists are attached to one or two teams from which less than 50% of the employment specialist's caseload is comprised.
	3	Employment specialists are attached to one or two mental health treatment teams, from which at least 50–74% of the employment specialist's caseload is comprised.
	4	Employment specialists are attached to one or two mental health treatment teams, from which at least 75–89% of the employment specialist's caseload is comprised.
	5	Employment specialists are attached to one or two mental health treatment teams, from which 90–100% of the employment specialist's caseload is comprised.

Directions: Circle one anchor number for each criterion.

Item Score:_____

ORGANIZATION

Criterion ②

Integration of rehabilitation with mental health treatment through frequent team member contact: Employment specialists actively participate in weekly mental health treatment team meetings (not replaced by administrative meetings) that discuss individual clients and their employment goals with shared decision-making. Employment specialist's office is in close proximity to (or shared with) their mental health treatment team members. Documentation of mental health treatment and employment services are integrated in a single client record. Employment specialists help the team think about employment for people who haven't yet been referred to supported employment services.

DATA SOURCE		ANCHOR
MIS, DOC, INT, OBS	1	One or none is present.
	2	Two are present.
	3	Three are present.
	4	Four are present.
	5	Five are present.

All five key components are present.

☐ Employment specialist attends weekly mental health treatment team meetings.

☐ Employment specialist participates actively in treatment team meetings with shared decision-making.

☐ Employment services documentation (i.e., vocational assessment/profile, employment plan, progress notes) is integrated into client's mental health treatment record.

☐ Employment specialist's office is in close proximity to (or shared with) the mental health treatment team members.

☐ Employment specialist helps the team think about employment for people who haven't yet been referred to supported employment services.

Directions: Circle one anchor number for each criterion.

Item Score: _____

ORGANIZATION

Criterion 3

Collaboration between employment specialists and vocational rehabilitation counselors: The employment specialists and VR counselors have frequent contact for the purpose of discussing shared clients and identifying potential referrals.

DATA SOURCE		ANCHOR
DOC, INT, OBS, ISP	1	Employment specialists and VR counselors have client-related contacts (phone, email, in person) less than quarterly to discuss shared clients and referrals. **OR** Employment specialists and VR counselors do not communicate.
	2	Employment specialists and VR counselors have client-related contacts (phone, email, in person) at least quarterly to discuss shared clients and referrals.
	3	Employment specialists and VR counselors have client-related contacts (phone, email, in-person) monthly to discuss shared clients and referrals.
	4	Employment specialists and VR counselors have scheduled, face-to-face meetings at least quarterly, **OR** have client-related contacts (phone, email, in person) weekly to discuss shared clients and referrals.
	5	Employment specialists and VR counselors have scheduled, face-to-face meetings at least monthly and have client-related contacts (phone, email, in person) weekly to discuss shared clients and referrals.

Directions: Circle one anchor number for each criterion.

Item Score:_____

ORGANIZATION

Criterion **4**

Vocational unit: At least 2 full-time employment specialists and a team leader compose the employment unit. They have weekly client-based group supervision following the supported employment model in which strategies are identified and job leads are shared. They provide coverage for each other's caseload when needed.

DATA SOURCE		ANCHOR
MIS, INT, OBS	1	Employment specialists are not part of a vocational unit.
	2	Employment specialists have the same supervisor but do not meet as a group. They do not provide backup services for each other's caseload.
	3	Employment specialists have the same supervisor and discuss clients with each other on a weekly basis. They provide backup services for each other's caseloads as needed. **OR** If a program is in a rural area where employment specialists are geographically separate with one employment specialist at each site, the employment specialists meet 2–3 times monthly with their supervisor by teleconference.
	4	At least 2 employment specialists and a team leader form an employment unit with 2–3 regularly scheduled meetings per month for client-based group supervision in which strategies are identified, job leads are shared, and clients are discussed. They provide coverage for each other's caseloads, when needed. **OR** If a program is in a rural area where employment specialists are geographically separate with one employment specialist at each site, the employment specialists meet 2–3 times per month with their supervisor in person or by teleconference, and mental health practitioners are available to help the employment specialist with activities such as taking someone to work or picking up job applications.
	5	At least 2 full-time employment specialists and a team leader form an employment unit with weekly client-based group supervision based on the supported employment model in which strategies are identified and job leads are shared. They provide coverage for each other's caseloads, when needed.

Directions: Circle one anchor number for each criterion.

Item Score:_____

ORGANIZATION

Criterion 5 — **Role of employment supervisor:** Supported employment unit is led by a supported employment team leader. Employment specialists' skills are developed and improved through outcome-based supervision. All five key roles of the employment supervisor are present.

DATA SOURCE		ANCHOR
MIS, INT, DOC, OBS	1	One or none is present.
	2	Two are present.
	3	Three are present.
	4	Four are present.
	5	Five are present.

Five key roles of the employment supervisor:

- ☐ One full-time equivalent (FTE) supervisor is responsible for no more than 10 employment specialists. The supervisor does not have other supervisory responsibilities. (Program leaders supervising fewer than 10 employment specialists may spend a percentage of time on other supervisory activities on a prorated basis. For example, an employment supervisor responsible for 4 employment specialists may be devoted to SE supervision half time.)

- ☐ Supervisor conducts weekly supported employment supervision designed to review client situations and identify new strategies and ideas to help clients in their work lives.

- ☐ Supervisor communicates with mental health treatment team leaders to ensure that services are integrated, to problem-solve programmatic issues (such as referral process or transfer of follow-along to mental health workers), and to be a champion for the value of work. Attends a meeting for each mental health treatment team on a quarterly basis.

- ☐ Supervisor accompanies employment specialists who are new or having difficulty with job development in the field monthly to improve skills by observing, modeling, and giving feedback on skills (e.g., meeting employers for job development).

- ☐ Supervisor reviews current client outcomes with employment specialists and sets goals to improve program performance at least quarterly.

Directions: Circle one anchor number for each criterion.

Item Score:_____

ORGANIZATION

Criterion **6**

Zero-exclusion criteria: All clients interested in working have access to supported employment services regardless of job readiness factors, substance abuse, symptoms, history of violent behavior, cognition impairments, treatment nonadherence, and personal presentation. These apply during supported employment services too. Employment specialists offer to help with another job when one has ended, regardless of the reason that the job ended or number of jobs held. If VR has screening criteria, the mental health agency does not use them to exclude anybody. Clients are not screened out formally or informally.

DATA SOURCE		ANCHOR
DOC, INT, OBS	1	There is a formal policy to exclude clients due to lack of job readiness (e.g., substance abuse, history of violence, low level of functioning, etc.) by employment staff, case managers, or other practitioners.
	2	Most clients are unable to access supported employment services due to perceived lack of job readiness (e.g., substance abuse, history of violence, low level of functioning, etc.).
	3	Some clients are unable to access supported employment services due to perceived lack of job readiness (e.g., substance abuse, history of violence, low level of functioning, etc.).
	4	No evidence of exclusion, formal or informal. Referrals are not solicited by a wide variety of sources. Employment specialists offer to help with another job when one has ended, regardless of the reason that the job ended or number of jobs held.
	5	All clients interested in working have access to supported employment services. Mental health practitioners encourage clients to consider employment, and referrals for supported employment are solicited by many sources. Employment specialists offer to help with another job when one has ended, regardless of the reason that the job ended or number of jobs held.

Directions: Circle one anchor number for each criterion.

Item Score:_____

ORGANIZATION

Criterion 7

Agency focus on competitive employment: Agency promotes competitive work through multiple strategies. Agency intake includes questions about interest in employment. Agency displays written postings (e.g., brochures, bulletin boards, posters) about employment and supported employment services. The focus should be with the agency programs that provide services to adults with severe mental illness. Agency supports ways for clients to share work stories with other clients and staff. Agency measures rate of competitive employment and shares this information with agency leadership and staff.

DATA SOURCE		ANCHOR
DOC, INT, OBS	1	One or none is present.
	2	Two are present.
	3	Three are present.
	4	Four are present.
	5	Five are present.

Agency promotes competitive work through multiple strategies:

☐ Agency intake includes questions about interest in employment.

☐ Agency includes questions about interest in employment on all annual (or semi-annual) assessment or treatment plan reviews.

☐ Agency displays written postings (e.g., brochures, bulletin boards, posters) about working and supported employment services in lobby and other waiting areas.

☐ Agency supports ways for clients to share work stories with other clients and staff (e.g., agency-wide employment recognition events, in-service training, peer support groups, agency newsletter articles, invited speakers at client treatment groups, etc.) at least twice a year.

☐ Agency measures rate of competitive employment on at least a quarterly basis and shares outcomes with agency leadership and staff.

Directions: Circle one anchor number for each criterion.

Item Score: _____

ORGANIZATION

Criterion 8

Executive team support for SE: Agency executive team members (e.g., CEO/executive director, chief operating officer, QA director, chief financial officer, clinical director, medical director, human resource director) assist with supported employment implementation and sustainability. All five key components of executive team support are present.

DATA SOURCE		ANCHOR
DOC, INT, OBS	1	One is present.
	2	Two are present.
	3	Three are present.
	4	Four are present.
	5	Five are present.

☐ Executive director and clinical director demonstrate knowledge regarding the principles of evidence-based supported employment.

☐ Agency QA process includes an explicit review of the SE program, or components of the program, at least every six months through the use of the Supported Employment Fidelity Scale or until achieving high fidelity, and at least yearly thereafter. Agency QA process uses the results of the fidelity assessment to improve SE implementation and sustainability.

☐ At least one member of the executive team actively participates at SE leadership team meetings (steering committee meetings) that occur at least every six months for high-fidelity programs and at least quarterly for programs that have not yet achieved high fidelity. *Steering committee* is defined as a diverse group of stakeholders charged with reviewing fidelity, program implementation, and the service delivery system. Committee develops written action plans aimed at developing or sustaining high-fidelity services.

☐ The agency CEO/executive director communicates how SE services support the mission of the agency and articulates clear and specific goals for SE and/or competitive employment to all agency staff during the first six months and at least annually thereafter (e.g., SE kickoff, all-agency meetings, agency newsletters, etc.). This item is not delegated to another administrator.

☐ SE program leader shares information about EBP barriers and facilitators with the executive team (including the CEO) at least twice each year. The executive team helps the program leader identify and implement solutions to barriers.

Directions: Circle one anchor number for each criterion.

Item Score:_____

SERVICES

Criterion **1**

Work incentives planning: All clients are offered assistance in obtaining comprehensive, individualized work incentives planning before starting a new job and assistance accessing work incentives planning thereafter when making decisions about changes in work hours and pay. Work incentives planning includes SSA benefits, medical benefits, medication subsidies, housing subsidies, food stamps, spouse and dependent children benefits, past job retirement benefits and any other source of income. Clients are provided information and assistance about reporting earnings to SSA, housing programs, VA programs, etc., depending on the person's benefits.

DATA SOURCE		ANCHOR
DOC, INT, OBS, ISP	1	Work incentives planning is not readily available or easily accessible to most clients served by the agency.
	2	Employment specialist gives client contact information about where to access information about work incentives planning.
	3	Employment specialist discusses with each client changes in benefits based on work status.
	4	Employment specialist or other MH practitioner offers clients assistance in obtaining comprehensive, individualized work incentives planning by a person trained in work incentives planning prior to clients starting a job.
	5	Employment specialist or other MH practitioner offers clients assistance in obtaining comprehensive, individualized work incentives planning by a specially trained work incentives planner prior to starting a job. They also facilitate access to work incentives planning when clients need to make decisions about changes in work hours and pay. Clients are provided information and assistance about reporting earnings to SSA, housing programs, etc., depending on the person's benefits.

Directions: Circle one anchor number for each criterion.

Item Score:_____

SERVICES

Criterion 2

Disclosure: Employment specialists provide clients with accurate information and assist with evaluating their choices to make an informed decision regarding what is revealed to the employer about having a disability.

DATA SOURCE		ANCHOR
DOC, INT, OBS	1	None is present.
	2	One is present.
	3	Two are present.
	4	Three are present.
	5	Four are present.

☐ Employment specialists do not require all clients to disclose their psychiatric disability at the work site in order to receive services.

☐ Employment specialists offer to discuss with clients the possible costs and benefits (pros and cons) of disclosure at the work site in advance of clients disclosing at the work site. Employment specialists describe how disclosure relates to requesting accommodations and the employment specialist's role communicating with the employer.

☐ Employment specialists discuss specific information to be disclosed (e.g., disclose receiving mental health treatment, or presence of a psychiatric disability, or difficulty with anxiety, or unemployed for a period of time, etc.) and offers examples of what could be said to employers.

☐ Employment specialists discuss disclosure on more than one occasion (e.g., if clients have not found employment after two months or if clients report difficulties on the job).

Directions: Circle one anchor number for each criterion.

Item Score:_____

SERVICES

Criterion ③

Ongoing, work-based vocational assessment: Initial vocational assessment occurs over 2–3 sessions and is updated with information from work experiences in competitive jobs. A vocational profile form that includes information about preferences, experiences, skills, current adjustment, strengths, personal contacts, etc., is updated with each new job experience. Aims at problem solving using environmental assessments and consideration of reasonable accommodations. Sources of information include the client, treatment team, clinical records, and, with the client's permission, family members and previous employers.

DATA SOURCE		ANCHOR
DOC, INT, OBS, ISP	1	Vocational evaluation is conducted prior to job placement with emphasis on office-based assessments, standardized tests, intelligence tests, work samples.
	2	Vocational assessment may occur through a stepwise approach that includes prevocational work experiences (e.g., work units in a day program), volunteer jobs, or set-aside jobs (e.g., NISH jobs, agency-run businesses, sheltered workshop jobs, affirmative businesses, enclaves).
	3	Employment specialists assist clients in finding competitive jobs directly without systematically reviewing interests, experiences, strengths, etc., and do not routinely analyze job loss (or job problems) for lessons learned.
	4	Initial vocational assessment occurs over 2–3 sessions in which interests and strengths are explored. Employment specialists help clients learn from each job experience and also work with the treatment team to analyze job loss, job problems, and job successes. They do not document these lessons learned in the vocational profile. **OR** The vocational profile is not updated on a regular basis.
	5	Initial vocational assessment occurs over 2–3 sessions and information is documented on a vocational profile form that includes preferences, experiences, skills, current adjustment, strengths, personal contacts, etc. The vocational profile form is used to identify job types and work environments. It is updated with each new job experience. Aims at problem solving using environmental assessments and consideration of reasonable accommodations. Sources of information include the client, treatment team, clinical records, and, with the client's permission, family members and previous employers. Employment specialists help clients learn from each job experience and also work with the treatment team to analyze job loss, job problems, and job successes.

Directions: Circle one anchor number for each criterion.

Item Score:_____

SERVICES

Criterion 4

Rapid job search for competitive job: Initial employment assessment and first face-to-face employer contact by the client or the employment specialist about a competitive job occurs within 30 days (1 month) after program entry.

DATA SOURCE		ANCHOR
DOC, INT, OBS, ISP	1	First face-to-face contact with an employer by the client or the employment specialist about a competitive job is on average 271 days or more (> 9 mos.) after program entry.
	2	First face-to-face contact with an employer by the client or the employment specialist about a competitive job is on average between 151 and 270 days (5–9 mos.) after program entry.
	3	First face-to-face contact with an employer by the client or the employment specialist about a competitive job is on average between 61 and 150 days (2–5 mos.) after program entry.
	4	First face-to-face contact with an employer by the client or the employment specialist about a competitive job is on average between 31 and 60 days (1–2 mos.) after program entry.
	5	The program tracks employer contacts and the first face-to-face contact with an employer by the client or the employment specialist about a competitive job is on average within 30 days (1 month) after program entry.

Directions: Circle one anchor number for each criterion.

Item Score:_____

SERVICES

Criterion **5**

Individualized job search: Employment specialists make employer contacts aimed at making a good job match based on clients' preferences (relating to what each person enjoys and their personal goals) and needs (including experience, ability, symptomatology, health, etc.) rather than the job market (i.e., those jobs that are readily available). An individualized job search plan is developed and updated with information from the vocational assessment/profile form and new job/educational experiences.

DATA SOURCE		ANCHOR
DOC, INT, OBS, ISP	1	Less than 25% of employer contacts by the employment specialist are based on job choices that reflect client's preferences, strengths, symptoms, etc., rather than the job market.
	2	25–49% of employer contacts by the employment specialist are based on job choices that reflect client's preferences, strengths, symptoms, etc., rather than the job market.
	3	50–74% of employer contacts by the employment specialist are based on job choices that reflect client's preferences, strengths, symptoms, etc., rather than the job market.
	4	75–89% of employer contacts by the employment specialist are based on job choices that reflect client's preferences, strengths, symptoms, etc., rather than the job market and are consistent with the current employment plan.
	5	Employment specialist makes employer contacts based on job choices that reflect client's preferences, strengths, symptoms, lessons learned from previous jobs, etc., 90–100% of the time rather than the job market and are consistent with the current employment/job search plan. When clients have limited work experience, employment specialists provide information about a range of job options in the community.

Directions: Circle one anchor number for each criterion.

Item Score:_____

SERVICES

Criterion 6

Job development—frequent employer contact: Each employment specialist makes at least 6 face-to-face employer contacts per week on behalf of clients looking for work. (Rate for each, then calculate average and use the closest scale point.) An employer contact is counted even when an employment specialist meets the same employer more than one time in a week, and when the client is present or not present. Client-specific and generic contacts are included. Employment specialists use a weekly tracking form to document employer contacts.

DATA SOURCE		ANCHOR
DOC, INT	1	Employment specialist makes fewer than 2 face-to-face employer contacts per week that are client-specific.
	2	Employment specialist makes 2 face-to-face employer contacts per week that are client-specific, **OR** does not have a process for tracking.
	3	Employment specialist makes 4 face-to-face employer contacts per week that are client-specific, and uses a tracking form that is reviewed by the SE supervisor on a monthly basis.
	4	Employment specialist makes 5 face-to-face employer contacts per week that are client-specific, and uses a tracking form that is reviewed by the SE supervisor on a weekly basis.
	5	Employment specialist makes 6 or more face-to-face employer contacts per week that are client-specific, or 2 employer contacts times the number of people looking for work when there are fewer than 3 people looking for work on their caseload (e.g., new program). In addition, employment specialist uses a tracking form that is reviewed by the SE supervisor on a weekly basis.

Directions: Circle one anchor number for each criterion.

Item Score:_____

SERVICES

Criterion 7

Job development—quality of employer contact: Employment specialists build relationships with employers through multiple visits in person that are planned to learn the needs of the employer, convey what the SE program offers to the employer, and describe client strengths that are a good match for the employer. (Rate for each employment specialist, then calculate average and use the closest scale point.)

DATA SOURCE		ANCHOR
DOC, INT, OBS	1	Employment specialist meets employer when helping client to turn in job applications. **OR** Employment specialist rarely makes employer contacts.
	2	Employment specialist contacts employers to ask about job openings and then shares these "leads" with clients.
	3	Employment specialist follows up on advertised job openings by introducing self, describing program, and asking employer to interview client.
	4	Employment specialist meets with employers in person whether or not there is a job opening, advocates for clients by describing strengths, and asks employers to interview clients.
	5	Employment specialist builds relationships with employers through multiple visits in person that are planned to learn the needs of the employer, convey what the SE program offers to the employer, describe client strengths that are a good match for the employer.

Directions: Circle one anchor number for each criterion.

Item Score:_____

SERVICES

Criterion **8**

Diversity of job types: Employment specialists assist clients in obtaining different types of jobs.

DATA SOURCE		ANCHOR
DOC, INT, OBS, ISP	1	Employment specialists assist clients in obtaining different types of jobs less than 50% of the time.
	2	Employment specialists assist clients in obtaining different types of jobs 50–59% of the time.
	3	Employment specialists assist clients in obtaining different types of jobs 60–69% of the time.
	4	Employment specialists assist clients in obtaining different types of jobs 70–84% of the time.
	5	Employment specialists assist clients in obtaining different types of jobs 85–100% of the time.

Directions: Circle one anchor number for each criterion.

Item Score:_____

SERVICES

Criterion **9**

Diversity of employers: Employment specialists assist clients in obtaining jobs with different employers.

DATA SOURCE		ANCHOR
DOC, INT, OBS, ISP	1	Employment specialists assist clients in obtaining jobs with different employers less than 50% of the time.
	2	Employment specialists assist clients in obtaining jobs with different employers 50–59% of the time.
	3	Employment specialists assist clients in obtaining jobs with different employers 60–69% of the time.
	4	Employment specialists assist clients in obtaining jobs with different employers 70–84% of the time.
	5	Employment specialists assist clients in obtaining jobs with different employers 85–100% of the time.

Directions: Circle one anchor number for each criterion.

Item Score:_____

SERVICES

Criterion **10**

Competitive jobs: Employment specialists provide competitive job options that have permanent status rather than temporary or time-limited status, e.g., TE (transitional employment positions). Competitive jobs pay at least minimum wage, are jobs that anyone can apply for, and are not set aside for people with disabilities. (Seasonal jobs and jobs from temporary agencies that other community members use are counted as competitive jobs.)

DATA SOURCE		ANCHOR
DOC, INT, OBS, ISP	1	Employment specialists provide options for permanent competitive jobs less than 64% of the time. **OR** There are fewer than 10 current jobs.
	2	Employment specialists provide options for permanent competitive jobs about 65–74% of the time.
	3	Employment specialists provide options for permanent competitive jobs about 75–84% of the time.
	4	Employment specialists provide options for permanent competitive jobs about 85–94% of the time.
	5	95% or more competitive jobs held by clients are permanent.

Directions: Circle one anchor number for each criterion.

Item Score:_____

SERVICES

Criterion 11

Individualized follow-along supports: Clients receive different types of support for working a job that are based on the job, client preferences, work history, needs, etc. Supports are provided by a variety of people, including treatment team members (e.g., medication changes, social skills training, encouragement), family, friends, co-workers (i.e., natural supports), and employment specialist. Employment specialist also provides employer support (e.g., educational information, job, accommodations) at client's request. Employment specialist offers help with career development, assistance with education, a more desirable job, or more preferred job duties.

DATA SOURCE		ANCHOR
DOC, INT, OBS, ISP	1	Most clients do not receive supports after starting a job.
	2	About half of the working clients receive a narrow range of supports provided primarily by the employment specialist.
	3	Most working clients receive a narrow range of supports that are provided primarily by the employment specialist.
	4	Clients receive different types of support for working a job that are based on the job, client preferences, work history, needs, etc. Employment specialist provides employer supports at the client's request.
	5	Clients receive different types of support for working a job that are based on the job, client preferences, work history, needs, etc. Employment specialist also provides employer support (e.g., educational information, job accommodations) at client's request. The employment specialist helps people move on to more preferable jobs and also helps people with school or certified training programs. The site provides examples of different types of support, including enhanced supports by treatment team members.

Directions: Circle one anchor number for each criterion.

Item Score:_____

SERVICES

Criterion ⑫

Time-unlimited follow-along supports: Employment specialists have face-to-face contact with clients within 1 week before starting a job, within 3 days after starting a job, weekly for the first month, and at least monthly for a year or more, on average, after working steadily, and as desired by clients. Clients are transitioned to step down job supports from a mental health worker following steady employment. Employment specialists contact clients within 3 days of learning about the job loss.

DATA SOURCE		ANCHOR
DOC, INT, OBS, ISP	1	Employment specialist does not meet face-to-face with the client after the first month of starting a job.
	2	Employment specialist has face-to-face contact with less than half of the working clients for at least 4 months after starting a job.
	3	Employment specialist has face-to-face contact with at least half of the working clients for at least 4 months after starting a job.
	4	Employment specialist has face-to-face contact with working clients weekly for the first month after starting a job and at least monthly for a year or more, on average, after working steadily, and as desired by clients.
	5	Employment specialist has face-to-face contact with clients within 1 week before starting a job, within 3 days after starting a job, weekly for the first month, and at least monthly for a year or more, on average, after working steadily and as desired by clients. Clients are transitioned to step down job supports from a mental health worker following steady employment. Employment specialist contacts clients within 3 days of hearing about the job loss.

Directions: Circle one anchor number for each criterion.

Item Score: _____

SERVICES

Criterion **13**

Community-based services: Employment services such as engagement, job finding, and follow-along supports are provided in natural community settings by all employment specialists. (Rate each employment specialist based on their *total* weekly scheduled work hours; then calculate the average and use the closest scale point.)

DATA SOURCE		ANCHOR
DOC, INT, OBS	1	Employment specialist spends 30% or less of total scheduled work hours in the community.
	2	Employment specialist spends 30–39% of total scheduled work hours in the community.
	3	Employment specialist spends 40–49% of total scheduled work hours in the community.
	4	Employment specialist spends 50–64% of total scheduled work hours in the community.
	5	Employment specialist spends 65% or more of total scheduled work hours in the community.

Directions: Circle one anchor number for each criterion.

Item Score:_____

SERVICES

Criterion 14

Assertive engagement and outreach by integrated treatment team: Service termination is not based on missed appointments or fixed time limits. Systematic documentation of outreach attempts. Engagement and outreach attempts made by integrated team members. Multiple home/community visits. Coordinated visits by employment specialist with integrated team member. Connect with family, when applicable. Once it is clear that the client no longer wants to work or continue SE services, the team stops outreach.

DATA SOURCE		ANCHOR
MIS, DOC, INT, OBS	1	Evidence that 2 or fewer strategies for engagement and outreach are used.
	2	Evidence that 3 strategies for engagement and outreach are used.
	3	Evidence that 4 strategies for engagement and outreach are used.
	4	Evidence that 5 strategies for engagement and outreach are used.
	5	Evidence that all 6 strategies for engagement and outreach are used: (i) Service termination is not based on missed appointments or fixed time limits. (ii) Systematic documentation of outreach attempts. (iii) Engagement and outreach attempts made by integrated team members. (iv) Multiple home/community visits. (v) Coordinated visits by employment specialist with integrated team member. (vi) Connect with family, when applicable.

Supported Employment Fidelity Scale Score Sheet

	STAFFING	
1.	Caseload size	Score:
2.	Employment services staff	Score:
3.	Vocational generalists	Score:
	ORGANIZATION	
1.	Integration of rehabilitation with mental health treatment through team assignment	Score:
2.	Integration of rehabilitation with mental health treatment through frequent team member contact	Score:
3.	Collaboration between employment specialists and vocational rehabilitation counselors	Score:
4.	Vocational unit	Score:
5.	Role of employment supervisor	Score:
6.	Zero-exclusion criteria	Score:
7.	Agency focus on competitive employment	Score:
8.	Executive team support for SE	Score:
	SERVICES	
1.	Work incentives planning	Score:
2.	Disclosure	Score:
3.	Ongoing, work-based vocational assessment	Score:
4.	Rapid job search for competitive job	Score:
5.	Individualized job search	Score:
6.	Job development—frequent employer contact	Score:
7.	Job development—quality of employer contact	Score:
8.	Diversity of job types	Score:
9.	Diversity of employers	Score:
10.	Competitive jobs	Score:
11.	Individualized follow-along supports	Score:
12.	Time-unlimited follow-along supports	Score:
13.	Community-based services	Score:
14.	Assertive engagement and outreach by integrated treatment team	Score:
	TOTAL:	

115–125 = Exemplary fidelity
100–114 = Good fidelity
74–99 = Fair fidelity
73 and below = Not supported employment

ACT Fidelity Scale and GOI Cover Sheet

Today's date: _____ / _____ / _____

Assessors' names: _____
_____
_____

Program name (or Program code): _____

Agency name: _____

Agency address:

_____
STREET

_____
CITY   STATE   ZIP CODE

Team leader or contact person: _____

Telephone: (____) ____–_____ E-mail: _____

Sources used for ACT fidelity and GOI assessments:

- ☐ Chart review (Number reviewed: _____)
- ☐ Brochure review
- ☐ Team meeting observation
- ☐ Supervision observation
- ☐ Team leader interview
- ☐ ACT team interviews (Number interviewed: _____)
- ☐ Consumer interviews (Number interviewed: _____)
- ☐ Family member interviews (Number interviewed: _____)
- ☐ Other staff interviewed (Number interviewed: _____)
- ☐ Other

ACT Fidelity Scale and GOI Cover Sheet ▸ PAGE 2 OF 2

Number of ACT team members: _____

Number of current ACT consumers: _____

Number of consumers served last year: _____

Funding source: _____

Agency location:
- ☐ Urban?
- ☐ Rural?

Date program was started: _____ / _____ / _____

ACT Fidelity Scale

Human resources: Structure and composition

CRITERION		1	2	3	4	5
H1	**Small caseload:** Consumer/provider ratio = 10:1	50 consumers/team member or more	35 – 49	21 – 34	11 – 20	10 consumers/team member or fewer
H2	**Team approach:** Provider group functions as team rather than as individual ACT team members; ACT team members know and work with all consumers	Less than 10% consumers with multiple team face-to-face contacts in reporting 2-week period	10 – 36%	37 – 63%	64 – 89%	90% or more consumers have face-to-face contact with >1 staff member in 2 weeks
H3	**Program meeting:** Meets often to plan and review services for each consumer	Service-planning for each consumer usually 1x/month or less	At least 2x/month but less often than 1x/week	At least 1x/week but less than 2x/week	At least 2x/week but less than 4x/week	Meets at least 4 days/week and reviews each consumer each time, even if only briefly
H4	**Practicing ACT leader:** Supervisor of Frontline ACT team members provides direct services	Supervisor provides no services	Supervisor provides services on rare occasions as backup	Supervisor provides services routinely as backup or less than 25% of the time	Supervisor normally provides services between 25% and 50% of the time	Supervisor provides services at least 50% of the time
H5	**Continuity of staffing:** Keeps same staffing over time	Greater than 80% turnover in 2 years	60 – 80% turnover in 2 years	40 – 59% turnover in 2 years	20 – 39% turnover in 2 years	Less than 20% turnover in 2 years
H6	**Staff capacity:** Operates at full staffing	Operated at less than 50% staffing in past 12 months	50 – 64%	65 – 79%	80 – 94%	Operated at 95% or more of full staffing in past 12 months
H7	**Psychiatrist on team:** At least 1 full-time psychiatrist for 100 consumers works with program	Less than .10 FTE regular psychiatrist for 100 consumers	.10 – .39 FTE for 100 consumers	.40 – .69 FTE for 100 consumers	.70 – .99 FTE for 100 consumers	At least 1 full-time psychiatrist assigned directly to 100-consumer program
H8	**Nurse on team:** At least 2 full-time nurses assigned for a 100-consumer program	Less than .20 FTE regular nurse for 100 consumers	.20 – .79 FTE for 100 consumers	.80 – 1.39 FTE for 100 consumers	1.40 – 1.99 FTE for 100 consumers	2 full-time nurses or more are members for 100-consumer program

continued

The Assertive Community Treatment Fidelity Scale appears courtesy of the Substance Abuse and Mental Health Services Administration. This document is in the public domain.

Human resources: Structure and composition continued

| | CRITERION | \multicolumn{5}{c}{RATINGS / ANCHORS} |
		1	2	3	4	5
H9	**Substance abuse specialist on team:** A 100-consumer program with at least 2 staff members with 1 year of training or clinical experience in substance abuse treatment	Less than .20 FTE S/A expertise for 100 consumers	.20 – .79 FTE for 100 consumers	.80 – 1.39 FTE for 100 consumers	1.40 – 1.99 FTE for 100 consumers	2 FTEs or more with 1 year S/A training or supervised S/A experience
H10	**Vocational specialist on team:** At least 2 team members with 1 year training/experience in vocational rehabilitation and support	Less than .20 FTE vocational expertise for 100 consumers	.20 – .79 FTE for 100 consumers	.80 – 1.39 FTE for 100 consumers	1.40 – 1.99 FTE for 100 consumers	2 FTEs or more with 1 year voc. rehab. training or supervised VR experience
H11	**Program size:** Of sufficient absolute size to consistently provide necessary staffing diversity and coverage	Less than 2.5 FTE staff	2.5 – 4.9 FTE	5.0 – 7.4 FTE	7.5 – 9.9 FTE	At least 10 FTE staff

Organizational boundaries

	CRITERION	RATINGS / ANCHORS				
		1	2	3	4	5
01	**Explicit admission criteria:** Has clearly identified mission to serve a particular population. Has and uses measurable and operationally defined criteria to screen out inappropriate referrals.	Has no set criteria and takes all types of cases as determined outside the program	Has a generally defined mission but admission process dominated by organizational convenience	Tries to seek and select a defined set of consumers but accepts most referrals	Typically actively seeks and screens referrals carefully but occasionally bows to organizational pressure	Actively recruits a defined population and all cases comply with explicit admission criteria
02	**Intake rate:** Takes consumers in at a low rate to maintain a stable service environment	Highest monthly intake rate in the last 6 months = greater than 15 consumers/month	13 – 15	10 – 12	7 – 9	Highest monthly intake rate in the last 6 months no greater than 6 consumers/month
03	**Full responsibility for treatment services:** In addition to case management, directly provides psychiatric services, counseling/psychotherapy, housing support, substance abuse treatment, employment and rehabilitative services	Provides no more than case management services	Provides 1 of 5 additional services and refers externally for others	Provides 2 of 5 additional services and refers externally for others	Provides 3 or 4 of 5 additional services and refers externally for others	Provides all 5 services to consumers
04	**Responsibility for crisis services:** Has 24-hour responsibility for covering psychiatric crises	Has no responsibility for handling crises after hours	Emergency service has program-generated protocol for program consumers	Is available by phone, mostly in consulting role	Provides emergency service backup; e.g., program is called, makes decision about need for direct program involvement	Provides 24-hour coverage
05	**Responsibility for hospital admissions:** Is involved in hospital admissions	Is involved in fewer than 5% decisions to hospitalize	ACT team is involved in 5% – 34% of admissions	ACT team is involved in 35% – 64% of admissions	ACT team is involved in 65% – 94% of admissions	ACT team is involved in 95% or more admissions

continued

Organizational boundaries continued

	CRITERION	RATINGS / ANCHORS				
		1	2	3	4	5
06	**Responsibility for hospital discharge planning:** Is involved in planning for hospital discharges	Is involved in fewer than 5% of hospital discharges	5% – 34% of program consumer discharges planned jointly with program	35% – 64% of program consumer discharges planned jointly with program	65 – 94% of program consumer discharges planned jointly with program	95% or more discharges planned jointly with program
07	**Time-unlimited services (graduation rate):** Rarely closes cases but remains the point of contact for all consumers as needed	More than 90% of consumers are expected to be discharged within 1 year	From 38 – 90% of consumers expected to be discharged within 1 year	From 18 – 37% of consumers expected to be discharged within 1 year	From 5 – 17% of consumers expected to be discharged within 1 year	All consumers served on a time-unlimited basis, with fewer than 5% expected to graduate annually

Nature of services

CRITERION		1	2	3	4	5
S1	**Community-based services:** Works to monitor status, develop community living skills in community rather than in office	Less than 20% of face-to-face contacts in community	20 – 39%	40 – 59%	60 – 79%	80% of total face-to-face contacts in community
S2	**No dropout policy:** Retains high percentage of consumers	Less than 50% of caseload retained over 12-month period	50 – 64%	65 – 79%	80 – 94%	95% or more of caseload is retained over a 12-month period
S3	**Assertive engagement mechanisms:** As part of ensuring engagement, uses street outreach and legal mechanisms (probation/parole, OP commitment) as indicated and as available	Passive in recruitment and re-engagement; almost never uses street outreach legal mechanisms	Makes initial attempts to engage but generally focuses on most motivated consumers	Tries outreach and uses legal mechanisms only as convenient	Usually has plan for engagement and uses most mechanisms available	Demonstrates consistently well-thought-out strategies and uses street outreach and legal mechanisms whenever appropriate
S4	**Intensity of service:** High total amount of service time, as needed	Average 15 minutes/week or less of face-to-face contact for each consumer	15 – 49 minutes/week	50 – 84 minutes/week	85 – 119 minutes/week	Average 2 hours/week or more of face-to-face contact for each consumer
S5	**Frequency of contact:** High number of service contacts, as needed	Average less than 1 face-to-face contact/week or fewer for each consumer	1 – 2x/week	2 – 3x/week	3 – 4x/week	Average 4 or more face-to-face contacts/week for each consumer
S6	**Work with informal support system:** With or without consumer present, provides support and skills for consumer's support network: family, landlords, employers	Less than .5 contact/month for each consumer with support system	.5 – 1 contact/month for each consumer with support system in the community	1 – 2 contacts/month for each consumer with support system in the community	2 – 3 contacts/month for consumer with support system in the community	4 or more contacts/month for each consumer with support system in the community
S7	**Individualized substance abuse treatment:** 1 or more team members provides direct treatment and substance abuse treatment for consumers with substance-use disorders	No direct, individualized substance abuse treatment provided	Team variably addresses SA concerns with consumers; provides no formal, individualized SA treatment	While team integrates some substance abuse treatment into regular consumer contact, no formal, individualized SA treatment	Some formal individualized SA treatment offered; consumers with substance-use disorders spend less than 24 minutes/week in such treatment	Consumers with substance-use disorders average 24 minutes/week or more in formal substance abuse treatment

continued

Nature of services continued

CRITERION		1	2	3	4	5
S8	**Co-occurring disorder treatment groups:** Uses group modalities as treatment strategy for consumers with substance-use disorders	Fewer than 5% of consumers with substance-use disorders attend at least 1 substance abuse treatment group meeting a month	5 – 19%	20 – 34%	35 – 49%	50% or more of consumers with substance-use disorders attend at least 1 substance abuse treatment group meeting/month
S9	**Dual Disorders (DD) Model:** Uses a non-confrontational, stage-wise treatment model, follows behavioral principles, considers interactions of mental illness and substance abuse, and has gradual expectations of abstinence	Fully based on traditional model: confrontation; mandated abstinence; higher power, etc.	Uses primarily traditional model: e.g., refers to AA; uses inpatient detox & rehab; recognizes need to persuade consumers in denial or who don't fit AA	Uses mixed model: e.g., DD principles in treatment plans; refers consumers to persuasion groups; uses hospitalization for rehab.; refers to AA, NA	Uses primarily DD model: e.g., DD principles in treatment plans; persuasion and active treatment groups; rarely hospitalizes for rehab. or detox except for medical necessity; refers out some SA treatment	Fully based in DD treatment principles, with treatment provided by ACT staff members
S10	**Role of consumers on treatment team:** Consumers involved as team members providing direct services	Consumers not involved in providing service	Consumers fill consumer-specific service roles (e.g., self-help)	Consumers work part-time in case-management roles with reduced responsibilities	Consumers work full-time in case management roles with reduced responsibilities	Consumers employed full-time as ACT team members (e.g., case managers) with full professional status

The Assertive Community Treatment Fidelity Scale appears courtesy of the Substance Abuse and Mental Health Services Administration. This document is in the public domain.

ACT Fidelity Score Sheet

Date of visit: _____ / _____ / _____

Agency name: _____

Assessors' names: _____

		Assessor 1	Assessor 2	Consensus
H1	Small caseload			
H2	Team approach			
H3	Program meeting			
H4	Practicing ACT leader			
H5	Continuity of staffing			
H6	Staff capacity			
H7	Psychiatrist on team			
H8	Nurse on team			
H9	Substance abuse specialist on team			
H10	Vocational specialist on team			
H11	Program size			
O1	Explicit admission criteria			
O2	Intake rate			
O3	Full responsibility for treatment services			
O4	Responsibility for crisis services			
O5	Responsibility for hospital admissions			
O6	Responsibility for hospital discharge planning			
O7	Time-unlimited services			
S1	Community-based services			
S2	No dropout policy			
S3	Assertive engagement mechanisms			
S4	Intensity of service			
S5	Frequency of contact			
S6	Work with support system			
S7	Individualized substance abuse treatment			
S8	Co-occurring disorder treatment groups			
S9	Dual Disorders (DD) Model			
S10	Role of consumers on treatment team			
Total mean score				

Illness Management and Recovery Fidelity Scale

STAFFING

CRITERIA

1. Number of people in a session or group: IMR is taught individually or in groups of 8 or fewer participants.

RATINGS/ANCHORS

1	2	3	4	5
Some sessions taught with more than 15 participants	Some sessions taught with 13–15 participants	Some sessions taught with 11–12 participants	Some sessions taught with 9–10 participants	All IMR sessions taught individually or in groups of 8 or fewer

CRITERIA

2. Program length: Participants receive at least 3 months of weekly IMR sessions or equivalent (for example, every 2 weeks for at least 6 months).

RATINGS/ANCHORS

1	2	3	4	5
Less than 20% of IMR participants receive at least 3 months of weekly sessions	20–39% of IMR participants receive at least 3 months of weekly sessions	40–69% of IMR participants receive at least 3 months of weekly sessions	70–89% of IMR participants receive at least 3 months of weekly sessions	At least 90% of IMR participants receive at least 3 months of weekly sessions

CRITERIA

3. Comprehensiveness of the curriculum:

- Recovery strategies
- Practical facts about mental illnesses
- Stress-vulnerability model
- Building social support
- Using medication effectively
- Drug and alcohol use
- Reducing relapses
- Coping with stress
- Coping with persistent symptoms
- Getting your needs met in the mental health system
- Healthy lifestyles

RATINGS/ANCHORS

1	2	3	4	5
Curriculum materials include only 1 topic OR Educational handouts are not available	Curriculum materials include 2 or 3 topic areas	Curriculum materials include 4 or 5 topic areas	Curriculum materials include 6 or 7 topic areas	Curriculum materials include 8 or more topic areas

continued on next page

STAFFING (continued)

CRITERIA
4. Provision of educational handouts: All participants receive IMR handouts.

RATINGS/ANCHORS				
1	2	3	4	5
Less than 20% of IMR participants receive educational handouts	20–39% of IMR participants receive educational handouts	40–69% of IMR participants receive educational handouts	70–89% of IMR participants receive educational handouts	At least 90% of IMR participants receive educational handouts

CRITERIA
5. Involvement of significant others:
- At least 1 IMR-related contact in the last month

  OR
- Involvement with the participant in pursuing goals (for example, helping with home practice assignments)

RATINGS/ANCHORS				
1	2	3	4	5
Less than 20% of IMR participants have significant others involved	20–29% of IMR participants have significant others involved	30–39% of IMR participants have significant others involved	40–49% of IMR participants have significant others involved	At least 50% of IMR participants have significant others involved

ASSIGNMENTS

CRITERIA
6. IMR goal setting:
- Realistic and measurable
- Individualized
- Pertinent to recovery process
- Linked to IMR plan

RATINGS/ANCHORS				
1	2	3	4	5
Less than 20% of IMR participants have at least 1 personal goal in their chart	20–39% of IMR participants have at least 1 personal goal in their chart	40–69% of IMR participants have at least 1 personal goal in their chart	70–89% of IMR participants have at least 1 personal goal in their chart	At least 90% of IMR participants have at least 1 personal goal in their chart

continued on next page

ASSIGNMENTS (continued)

CRITERIA

7. IMR goal follow-up: Practitioners and participants collaboratively follow up on goals.

RATINGS/ANCHORS

1	2	3	4	5
Less than 20% of IMR participants have follow-up on goals documented in their chart	20–39% of IMR participants have follow-up on goals documented in their chart	40–69% of IMR participants have follow-up on goals documented in their chart	70–89% of IMR participants have follow-up on goals documented in their chart	At least 90% of IMR participants have follow-up on goals documented in their chart

CRITERIA

8. Motivation-based strategies:
- New information and skills
- Positive perspectives
- Pros and cons of change
- Hope and self-efficacy

RATINGS/ANCHORS

1	2	3	4	5
Less than 20% of IMR sessions use at least 1 motivation-based strategy	20–29% of IMR sessions use at least 1 motivation-based strategy	30–39% of IMR sessions use at least 1 motivation-based strategy	40–49% of IMR sessions use at least 1 motivation-based strategy	At least 50% of IMR sessions use at least 1 motivation-based strategy

CRITERIA

9. Educational techniques:
- Interactive teaching
- Checking for understanding
- Breaking down information
- Reviewing information

RATINGS/ANCHORS

1	2	3	4	5
Less than 20% of IMR sessions use at least 1 educational technique	20–29% of IMR sessions use at least 1 educational technique	30–39% of IMR sessions use at least 1 educational technique	40–49% of IMR sessions use at least 1 educational technique	At least 50% of IMR sessions use at least 1 educational technique

continued on next page

ASSIGNMENTS (continued)

CRITERIA

10. Cognitive-behavioral techniques:
- Reinforcement
- Shaping
- Modeling
- Role playing
- Cognitive restructuring
- Relaxation training

RATINGS/ANCHORS

1	2	3	4	5
Less than 20% of IMR sessions use at least 1 cognitive-behavioral technique	20–29% of IMR sessions use at least 1 cognitive-behavioral technique	30–39% of IMR sessions use at least 1 cognitive-behavioral technique	40–49% of IMR sessions use at least 1 cognitive-behavioral technique	At least 50% of IMR sessions use at least 1 cognitive-behavioral technique

CRITERIA

11. Coping skills training:
- Review current coping
- Amplify current coping or develop new coping skills
- Behavioral rehearsal
- Review effectiveness
- Modify as necessary

RATINGS/ANCHORS

1	2	3	4	5
Few or none of the practitioners are familiar with the principles of coping skills training	Some of the practitioners are familiar with the principles of coping skills training, with a low level of use	Some of the practitioners are familiar with the principles of coping skills training, with a moderate level of use	The majority of practitioners are familiar with the principles of coping skills training and use it regularly	All practitioners are familiar with the principles of coping skills training and use it regularly

CRITERIA

12. Relapse prevention training:
- Identify triggers
- Identify early warning signs
- Stress management
- Ongoing monitoring
- Rapid intervention as needed

RATINGS/ANCHORS

1	2	3	4	5
Few or none of the practitioners are familiar with the principles of relapse prevention training	Some of the practitioners are familiar with the principles of relapse prevention training, with a low level of use	Some of the practitioners are familiar with the principles of relapse prevention training, with a moderate level of use	The majority of the practitioners are familiar with the principles of relapse prevention training and use it regularly	All practitioners are familiar with the principles of relapse prevention training and use it regularly, as documented by relapse prevention plans in participants' charts

continued on next page

ASSIGNMENTS (continued)

CRITERIA

13. Behavioral tailoring for medication:
Behavioral tailoring includes developing strategies tailored to each participant's needs, motives, and resources (for example, choosing medication that requires less frequent dosing and placing medication next to one's toothbrush).

RATINGS/ANCHORS

1	2	3	4	5
Few or none of the practitioners are familiar with the principles of behavioral tailoring for medication	Some of the practitioners are familiar with the principles of behavioral tailoring for medication, with a low level of use	Some of the practitioners are familiar with the principles of behavioral tailoring for medication, with a moderate level of use	The majority of the practitioners are familiar with the principles of behavioral tailoring for medication and use it regularly	All practitioners are familiar with the principles of behavioral tailoring for medication and either teach or reinforce it regularly

Illness Management and Recovery Fidelity Scale Score Sheet

Agency name: _____

Date of visit: _____ / _____ / _____

Assessors' names: _____

_____

	Program Element	Assessor 1	Assessor 2	Consensus
1	Number of people in a session or group			
2	Program length			
3	Comprehensiveness of the curriculum			
4	Provision of educational handouts			
5	Involvement of significant others			
6	IMR goal setting			
7	IMR goal follow-up			
8	Motivation-based strategies			
9	Educational techniques			
10	Cognitive-behavioral techniques			
11	Coping skills training			
12	Relapse prevention training			
13	Behavioral tailoring for medication			
	Total mean score			

Contents of the CD-ROM

Implementing Evidence-Based Practices: An Agency's Tasks

Table 6: Implementation Measures

Implementation Task Checklists

Measurement Tools, Fidelity Scales

Measures of State Agency/Governmental or Funder Leadership

State Health Authority Yardstick: The SHAY Rating Scale

Measures of Organizational Readiness

Agency Readiness for IPS Supported Employment Checklist

Measures of Practice Sustainability

Dartmouth Sustainability Interview Template: A Guide for Interviewing IPS Team Leader

Agency/Administrative Fidelity Assessment Tools

GOI Cover Sheet

GOI Fidelity Scale

GOI Score Sheet

Dual Diagnosis Capability in Addiction Treatment (DDCAT) Toolkit

Dual Diagnosis Capability in Mental Health Treatment (DDCMHT) Toolkit

Dual Diagnosis Capability in Health Care Settings (DDCHCS)

Fidelity Scales and Protocols for Programs

Supported Employment Fidelity Scale (2008, Dartmouth version)

Supported Employment Fidelity Scale Score Sheet

IDDT Fidelity Scale and Protocol (found in *Integrated Treatment for Co-Occurring Disorders: Evaluating Your Program*)

IDDT Fidelity Scale Cover Sheet

IDDT Fidelity Scale

IDDT Fidelity Scale Score Sheet

Illness Management and Recovery Fidelity Scale Protocol

Contents of the CD-ROM

Illness Management and Recovery Fidelity Scale with Score Sheet

Illness Management and Recovery Treatment Integrity Scale (IT-IS)

ACT Fidelity Scale and Protocol (found in *Assertive Community Treatment: Evaluating Your Program*)

Tool for Measurement of Assertive Community Treatment (TMACT) Summary Scale

MedTEAM Fidelity Scale, Chart, and Protocol (found in *MedTEAM: Evaluating Your Program*)

Family Psychoeducation Fidelity Scale and Protocol (found in *Family Psychoeducation: Evaluating Your Program*)

References

Introduction

Balas, E. A., and S. A. Boren. 2000. "Managing Clinical Knowledge for Health Care Improvement." In *Yearbook of Medical Informatics 2000: Patient-Centered Systems,* edited by J. Bemmel and A. T. McCray, 65–70. Stuttgart, Germany: Schattauer.

Fox, L., R. E. Drake, K. T. Mueser, M. F. Brunette, D. R. Becker, M. McGovern, D. Cimpean, S. J. Bartels, W. C. Torrey, F. P. Foster, D. A. Strickler, M. R. Merrens, and S. C. Acquilano. 2010. *Integrated Dual Disorders Treatment: Best Practices, Skills, and Resources for Successful Client Care.* Center City, MN: Hazelden.

Gawande, A. 2012. "Big Med." *The New Yorker,* Aug. 13 and 20, 52–63.

Green, L. W., J. M. Ottoson, C. Garcia, and R. A. Hiatt. 2009. "Diffusion Theory and Knowledge Dissemination, Utilization, and Integration in Public Health." *Annual Review of Public Health* 30:151–74.

Institute of Medicine. 2001. *Crossing the Quality Chasm: A New Health System for the 21st Century.* Washington, DC: National Academy Press.

Lehman, A. F., and D. M. Steinwachs. 1998. "Patterns of Usual Care for Schizophrenia: Initial Results from the Schizophrenia Patient Outcomes Research Team (PORT) Client Survey." *Schizophrenia Bulletin* 24: 11–23.

Longtin, Y., H. Sax, B. Allegranzi, F. Schneider, and D. Pittet. Mar. 31, 2011. "Hand Hygiene." *New England Journal of Medicine* 364 (13): e24.

President's New Freedom Commission on Mental Health. 2003. *Achieving the Promise: Transforming Mental Health Care in America.* DHHS Publication No. SMA-03-3832. Rockville, MD.

Chapter 2

Aarons, G. A. 2004. "Mental Health Provider Attitudes toward Adoption of Evidence-Based Practice: The Evidence-Based Practice Attitude Scale (EBPAS)." *Mental Health Services Research* 6:61–74.

AIMS Center. 2011. "Step 3: Team Building." Seattle, WA: Advancing Integrated Mental Health Solutions, University of Washington. Retrieved Nov. 27, 2011. http://uwaims.org/implementation-tools.html.

Becker, D. R., R. E. Drake, and G. R. Bond. 2011. "Benchmark Outcomes in Supported Employment." *American Journal of Psychiatric Rehabilitation* 14:230–36.

Becker, D. R., R. E. Drake, G. R. Bond, S. Nawaz, W. R. Haslett, and R. A. Martinez. 2011. "A National Mental Health Learning Collaborative on Supported Employment." *Psychiatric Services* 62:704–6.

Becker, D. R., S. Swanson, G. R. Bond, and M. R. Merrens. 2011. *Evidence-Based Supported Employment Fidelity Review Manual.* 2nd ed. Lebanon, NH: Dartmouth Psychiatric Research Center.

References

Becker, D. R., S. J. Swanson, G. R. Bond, L. Carlson, L. Flint, G. Smith, and D. Lynde. 2008. *Supported Employment Fidelity Scale.* Unpublished scale. Lebanon, NH: Dartmouth Psychiatric Research Center. http://dms.dartmouth.edu/prc/employment/.

Bond, G. R., R. E. Drake, C. A. Rapp, G. J. McHugo, and H. Xie. 2009. "Individualization and Quality Improvement: Two New Scales to Complement Measurement of Program Fidelity." *Administration and Policy in Mental Health and Mental Health Services Research* 36:349–57.

Bond, G. R., G. J. McHugo, D. R. Becker, A. E. Peterson, and R. E. Drake. 2012. *Dartmouth Sustainability Interview* (revised Feb. 29, 2012). Lebanon, NH: Dartmouth Psychiatric Research Center.

Bond, G. R., A. E. Peterson, D. R. Becker, and R. E. Drake. 2012. "Validating the Revised Individual Placement and Support Fidelity Scale (IPS-25)." *Psychiatric Services* 63:758–63.

Bond, G. R., J. Williams, L. Evans, M. Salyers, H. W. Kim, H. Sharpe, and H. S. Leff. 2000. *Psychiatric Rehabilitation Fidelity Toolkit.* Cambridge, MA: Human Services Research Institute.

Borntrager, C. F., B. F. Chorpita, C. Higa-McMillan, and J. R. Weisz. 2009. "Provider Attitudes toward Evidence-Based Practices: Are the Concerns with the Evidence or with the Manuals?" *Psychiatric Services* 60:677–81.

Bowen, S. K., R. P. Saunders, D. L. Richter, J. Hussey, K. Elder, and L. Lindley. 2010. "Assessing Levels of Adaptation during Implementation of Evidence-Based Interventions: Introducing the Rogers–Rütten Framework." *Health Science and Behavior* 37:815–30. http://heb.sagepub.com/content/837/816/815.full.pdf.

Carroll, K. M., C. Nich, R. L. Sifry, K. F. Nuro, T. L. Frankforter, S. A. Ball, L. Fenton, and B. J. Rounsaville. 2000. "A General System for Evaluating Therapist Adherence and Competence in Psychotherapy Research in the Addictions." *Drug and Alcohol Dependence* 57:225–38.

Finnerty, M. T., C. A. Rapp, G. R. Bond, D. W. Lynde, V. J. Ganju, and H. H. Goldman. 2009. "The State Health Authority Yardstick (SHAY)." *Community Mental Health Journal* 45: 228–36.

Frey, W. D., R. E. Drake, G. R. Bond, A. L. Miller, H. H. Goldman, D. S. Salkever, and S. Holsenbeck. 2011. *Mental Health Treatment Study: Final Report to Social Security Administration.* Rockville, MD: Westat. http://socialsecurity.gov/disabilityresearch/mentalhealth.htm.

Gotham, H. J., R. E. Claus, K. Selig, and A. L. Homer. 2010. "Increasing Program Capability to Provide Treatment for Co-occurring Substance Use and Mental Disorders: Organizational Characteristics." *Journal of Substance Abuse Treatment* 38:160–69.

Howard, P. B., P. El-Mallakh, A. L. Miller, M. K. Rayens, G. R. Bond, K. Henderson, and A. T. Cooley. 2009. "Prescriber Fidelity to a Medication Management Evidence-Based Practice in the Treatment of Schizophrenia." *Psychiatric Services* 60:929–35.

Martino, S., S. A. Ball, C. Nich, T. L. Frankforter, and K. M. Carroll. 2008. "Community Program Therapist Adherence and Competence in Motivational Enhancement Therapy." *Drug and Alcohol Dependence* 96:37–48.

Massatti, R. R., H. A. Sweeney, P. C. Panzano, and D. Roth. 2008. "The De-adoption of Innovative Mental Health Practices (IMHP): Why Organizations Choose Not to Sustain an IMHP." *Administration and Policy in Mental Health and Mental Health Services Research* 35:50–65.

McGovern, M. P., A. L. Matzkin, and J. Giard. 2007. "Assessing the Dual Diagnosis Capability of Addiction Treatment Services: The Dual Diagnosis Capability in Addiction Treatment (DDCAT) Index." *Journal of Dual Diagnosis* 3:111–23.

McGuire, A. B., L. G. Stull, K. Mueser, M. Santos, A. Mook, C. Nicksic, N. Rose, L. White, and M. P. Salyers. 2012. "Development and Reliability of an Illness Management and Recovery Clinical Competence Measure." *Psychiatric Services* 63:772–78.

McHugo, G. J., R. E. Drake, R. Whitley, G. R. Bond, K. Campbell, C. A. Rapp, H. H. Goldman, W. J. Lutz, and M. T. Finnerty. 2007. "Fidelity Outcomes in the National Implementing Evidence-Based Practices Project." *Psychiatric Services* 58:1279–84.

Monroe-DeVita, M., G. B. Teague, and L. L. Moser. 2011. "The TMACT: A New Tool for Measuring Fidelity to Assertive Community Treatment." *Journal of the American Psychiatric Nurses Association* 17:17–29.

Mueser, K. T., S. Gingerich, G. R. Bond, K. Campbell, and J. Williams. 2005. "Illness Management and Recovery Fidelity Scale" (revised Feb. 24, 2005). In *Illness Management and Recovery Implementation Resource Kit,* edited by K. T. Mueser and S. Gingerich. Rockville, MD: Center for Mental Health Services, Substance Abuse and Mental Health Services Administration.

Panzano, P. C., and D. Roth. 2006. "The Decision to Adopt Evidence-Based and Other Innovative Mental Health Practices: Risky Business?" *Psychiatric Services* 57:1153–61.

Proctor, E., H. Silmere, R. Raghavan, P. Hovmand, G. Aarons, A. Bunger, R. Griffey, and M. Hensley. 2011. "Outcomes for Implementation Research: Conceptual Distinctions, Measurement Challenges, and Research Agenda." *Administration and Policy in Mental Health and Mental Health Services Research* 38:65–76.

Resnick, S. G., and R. A. Rosenheck. 2009. "Scaling Up the Dissemination of Evidence-Based Mental Health Practice to Large Systems and Long-Term Time Frames." *Psychiatric Services* 60:682–85.

Rogers, E. M. 2003. *Diffusion of Innovations.* 5th ed. New York: Free Press.

SAMHSA. 2010. *MedTEAM (Medication Treatment, Evaluation, and Management) Evidence-Based Practices (EBP) Kit* (HHS Pub. No. SMA10-4549). Rockville, MD: Center for Mental Health Services, Substance Abuse and Mental Health Services Administration, U.S. Department of Health and Human Services. http://store.samhsa.gov/shin/content//SMA10-4549/EvaluatingYourProgram-MT.pdf.

Swain, K., R. Whitley, G. J. McHugo, and R. E. Drake. 2010. "The Sustainability of Evidence-Based Practices in Routine Mental Health Agencies." *Community Mental Health Journal* 46:119–29.

Swanson, S. J., and D. R. Becker. 2011. *Agency Readiness for IPS Supported Employment Checklist.* Lebanon, NH: Dartmouth Psychiatric Research Center.

Taylor, A. C., G. R. Bond, J. Tsai, P. B. Howard, P. El-Mallakh, M. Finnerty, E. Kealey, B. Myrhol, K. Kalk, N. Adams, and A. L. Miller. 2009. "A Scale to Evaluate Quality of Medication Management: Development and Psychometric Properties." *Administration and Policy in Mental Health and Mental Health Services Research* 36:247–54.

Teague, G. B., G. R. Bond, and R. E. Drake. 1998. "Program Fidelity in Assertive Community Treatment: Development and Use of a Measure." *American Journal of Orthopsychiatry* 68:216–32.

References

Torrey, W. C., G. R. Bond, G. J. McHugo, and K. Swain. 2012. "Evidence-Based Practice Implementation in Community Mental Health Settings: The Relative Importance of Key Domains of Implementation Activity." *Administration and Policy in Mental Health and Mental Health Services Research* 39:353–64.

Tsai, J., & G. R. Bond. 2008. "A Comparison of Electronic Medical Records to Conventional Paper Records in Community Mental Health Centers." *International Journal for Quality in Health Care* 20:136–43.

Chapter 4

Fox, L., R. E. Drake, K. T. Mueser, M. F. Brunette, D. R. Becker, M. McGovern, D. Cimpean, S. J. Bartels, W. C. Torrey, F. P. Foster, D. A. Strickler, M. R. Merrens, and S. C. Acquilano. 2010. *Integrated Dual Disorders Treatment: Best Practices, Skills, and Resources for Successful Client Care.* Center City, MN: Hazelden.

Gingerich, S., and K. T. Mueser. 2011. *Illness Management and Recovery: Personalized Skills and Strategies for Those with Mental Illness.* Center City, MN: Hazelden.

Morse, G., and M. McKasson. 2005. "Assertive Community Treatment." In *Evidence-Based Mental Practice: A Textbook,* edited by R. E. Drake, M. R. Merrens, and D. W. Lynde. New York: W.W. Norton.

Murray-Swank, A., and L. Dixon. 2005. "Evidence-Based Practices for Families of Individuals with Severe Mental Illness." In *Evidence-Based Mental Practice: A Textbook,* edited by R. E. Drake, M. R. Merrens, and D. W. Lynde. New York: W.W. Norton.

Swanson, S. J., and D. R. Becker. 2011. *Supported Employment: Applying the Individual Placement and Support (IPS) Model to Help Clients Compete in the Workforce.* Center City, MN: Hazelden.

Tsemberis, S. 2010. *Housing First: The Pathways Model to End Homelessness for People with Mental Illness and Addiction.* Center City, MN: Hazelden.

Chapter 5

Balas, E. A., and S. A. Boren. 2000. "Managing Clinical Knowledge for Health Care Improvement." In *Yearbook of Medical Informatics 2000: Patient-Centered Systems,* edited by J. Bemmel and A. T. McCray, 65–70. Stuttgart, Germany: Schattauer Verlagsgesellschaft mbH.

Green, L. W., J. M. Ottoson, C. Garcia, and R. A. Hiatt. 2009. "Diffusion Theory and Knowledge Dissemination, Utilization, and Integration in Public Health." *Annual Review of Public Health* 30:151–74

Rogers, E. M. 2003. *Diffusion of Innovations.* 5th ed. New York: Free Press.

Recommended Reading and Resources

■ ■ ■

Introduction

Drake, R. E., M. R. Merrens, and D. W. Lynde. *Evidence-Based Mental Health Practice: A Textbook.* 1st ed. New York: W.W. Norton, 2005.

Chapter 1

Articles Related to the National Implementing Evidence-Based Practices Project

GENERAL PAPERS

Isett, K. R., M. A. Burnman, B. Coleman-Beattie, P. A. Hyde, J. P. Morrissey, J. Magnabosco, C. A. Rapp, V. Ganju, and H. H. Goldman. "Implementation Issues for Evidence-Based Practices: The State Policy Context." *Psychiatric Services* 58 (2007): 914–21.

McHugo, G. J., R. E. Drake, R. Whitley, G. R. Bond, K. Campbell, C. A. Rapp, H. H. Goldman, W. T. Lutz, and M. T. Finnerty. "Fidelity Outcomes in the National Implementing Evidence-Based Practices Project." *Psychiatric Services* 58 (2007): 1279–84.

Swain, K., R. Whitley, G. J. McHugo, and R. E. Drake. "The Sustainability of Evidence-Based Practices in Routine Mental Health Agencies." *Community Mental Health Journal* 46 (2010): 119–129.

Torrey, W. C., D. W. Lynde, and P. Gorman. "Promoting the Implementation of Practices That Are Supported by Research: The National Implementing Evidence-Based Practices Project." *Child and Adolescent Psychiatric Clinics of North America* 14 (2005): 297–306.

PAPERS ON SPECIFIC EVIDENCE-BASED PRACTICES

Brunette, M. A., D. Asher, R. Whitley, W. J. Lutz, B. L. Wieder, A. M. Jones, and G. J. McHugo. "Implementation of Integrated Dual Disorders Treatment: A Qualitative Analysis of Facilitators and Barriers." *Psychiatric Services* 59 (2008): 989–95.

Mancini, A. D., L. L. Moser, R. Whitley, G. J. McHugo, G. R. Bond, M. T. Finnerty, and B. J. Burns. "Assertive Community Treatment: Facilitators and Barriers to Implementation in Routine Mental Health Settings." *Psychiatric Services* 60, no. 2 (2009): 189–95.

Marshall, T., C. A. Rapp, D. R. Becker, and G. R. Bond. "Key Factors for Implementing Supported Employment." *Psychiatric Services* 59 (2008): 886–92.

Whitley, R., S. Gingerich, W. J. Lutz, and K. T. Mueser. "Implementing the Illness Management and Recovery Program in Community Mental Health Settings: Facilitators and Barriers." *Psychiatric Services* 60 (2009): 202–9.

Implementation Manuals and Toolkits

Brunette, M. F., and other faculty from the Dartmouth Medical School. *Medication Management.* Co-occurring Disorders Program. Center City, MN: Hazelden, 2008.

Burns, B., and S. Phillips, eds. *Assertive Community Treatment Implementation Resource Kit.* Rockville, MD: Center for Mental Health Services, Substance Abuse and Mental Health Services Administration, 2002. (The 2008 version of this publication is available at http://store.samhsa.gov/product/Assertive-Community-Treatment-ACT-Evidence-Based-Practices-EBP-KIT/SMA08-4345.)

Fox, L., R. E. Drake, K. T. Mueser, M. F. Brunette, D. R. Becker, M. McGovern, D. Cimpean, S. J. Bartels, W. C. Torrey, F. P. Foster, D. A. Strickler, M. R. Merrens, and S. C. Acquilano. *Integrated Dual Disorders Treatment: Best Practices, Skills, and Resources for Successful Client Care.* Center City, MN: Hazelden, 2010.

Gingerich, S., and K. T. Mueser. *Illness Management and Recovery: Personalized Skills and Strategies for Those with Mental Illness.* Updated, revised ed. Center City, MN: Hazelden, 2011.

McFarlane, W., and L. Dixon, eds. *Family Psycho-education Implementation Resource Kit.* Rockville, MD: Center for Mental Health Services, Substance Abuse and Mental Health Services Administration, 2002. (The 2010 version of this publication is available at http://store.samhsa.gov/product/Family-Psychoeducation-Evidence-Based-Practices-KIT/SMA09-4423.)

McGovern, M., and other faculty from the Dartmouth Medical School. *Cognitive-Behavioral Therapy.* Co-occurring Disorders Program. Center City, MN: Hazelden, 2008.

McGovern, M., and other faculty from the Dartmouth Medical School. *Integrating Combined Therapies.* Co-occurring Disorders Program. Center City, MN: Hazelden, 2008.

Mueser, K. T., and other faculty from the Dartmouth Medical School. *Family Program.* Co-occurring Disorders Program. Center City, MN: Hazelden, 2008.

Swanson, S. J., and D. R. Becker. *Supported Employment: Applying the Individual Placement and Support (IPS) Model to Help Clients Compete in the Workforce.* Center City, MN: Hazelden, 2011.

Tsemberis, S. *Housing First Manual: The Pathways Model to End Homelessness for People with Mental Illness and Addiction.* Center City, MN: Hazelden, 2010.

Readings on Implementation Science

Damschroder, L. J., D. C. Aron, R. E. Keith, S. R. Kirsh, J. A. Alexander, and J. C. Lowery. "Fostering Implementation of Health Services Research Findings into Practice: A Consolidated Framework for Advancing Implementation Science." *Implementation Science* (IS) 4, no. 50 (2009). PubMed Central (PMC2736161).

Damschroder, L. J., and H. J. Hagedorn. "A Guiding Framework and Approach for Implementation Research in Substance Use Disorders Treatment." *Psychology of Addictive Behaviors* 25, no. 2 (2011): 194–205.

Ducharme, L. J., H. L. Mello, P. M. Roman, H. K. Knudsen, and J. A. Johnson. "Service Delivery in Substance Abuse Treatment: Reexamining 'Comprehensive' Care." *The Journal of Behavioral Health Services & Research* 34, no. 2 (2007): 121–36.

Garner, B. R. "Research on the Diffusion of Evidence-Based Treatments within Substance Abuse Treatment: A Systematic Review." *Journal of Substance Abuse Treatment* 36, no. 4 (2009): 376–99. PubMed Central (PMC2695403).

Glasgow, R. E. "RE-AIMing Research for Application: Ways to Improve Evidence for Family Medicine." *Journal of the American Board of Family Medicine (JABFM)* 19, no. 1 (2006): 11–19.

Institute of Medicine. *Crossing the Quality Chasm: A New Health System for the 21st Century.* Washington, DC: National Academy Press, 2001.

Manuel, J. K., H. J. Hagedorn, and J. W. Finney. "Implementing Evidence-Based Psychosocial Treatment in Specialty Substance Use Disorder Care." *Psychology of Addictive Behaviors* 25, no. 2 (2011): 225–37. PubMed Central (PMC3119356).

McKibbon, K. A., C. Lokker, N. L. Wilczynski, D. Ciliska, M. Dobbins, D. A. Davis, R. B. Haynes, and S. E. Straus. "A Cross-Sectional Study of the Number and Frequency of Terms Used to Refer to Knowledge Translation in a Body of Health Literature in 2006: A Tower of Babel?" *Implementation Science (IS)* 5, no. 16 (2010). PubMed Central (PMC2834600).

Powell, B. J., J. C. McMillen, E. K. Proctor, C. R. Carpenter, R. T. Griffey, A. C. Bunger, J. E. Glass, and J. L. York. "A Compilation of Strategies for Implementing Clinical Innovations in Health and Mental Health." *Medical Care Research and Review (MCRR)* 69, no. 2 (2012): 123–57.

Proctor, E., H. Silmere, R. Raghavan, P. Hovmand, G. Aarons, A. Bunger, R. Griffey, and M. Hensley. 2011. "Outcomes for Implementation Research: Conceptual Distinctions, Measurement Challenges, and Research Agenda." *Administration and Policy in Mental Health* 38, no. 2 (2011): 65–76. PubMed Central (PMC3068522).

Chapter 5

Brownson, R. C., G. A. Colditz, and E. K. Proctor, eds. *Dissemination and Implementation Research in Health: Translating Science to Practice.* New York: Oxford University Press, 2012.

Damschroder, L. J., D. C. Aron, R. E. Keith, S. R. Kirsh, J. A. Alexander, and J. C. Lowery. "Fostering Implementation of Health Services Research Findings into Practice: A Consolidated Framework for Advancing Implementation Science." *Implementation Science (IS)* 4, no. 50 (2009). PubMed Central (PMC2736161).

Fixsen, D. L., S. F. Naoom, K. A. Blasé, R. M. Friedman, and F. Wallace. *Implementation Research: A Synthesis of the Literature.* Tampa, FL: National Implementation Research Network, University of South Florida, 2005.

Glasgow, R. E., T. M. Bogt, and S. M. Boles. "Evaluating the Public Health Impact of Health Promotion Interventions: The RE-AIM Framework." *American Journal of Public Health* 89 (1999): 1322–27.

Manuel, J. K., H. J. Hagedorn, and J. W. Finney. "Implementing Evidence-Based Psychosocial Treatment in Specialty Substance Use Disorder Care." *Psychology of Addictive Behaviors* 25 (2011): 225–37.

McGovern, M. P., C. Lambert-Harris, G. J. McHugo, J. Giard, and L. Mangrum. "Improving the Dual Diagnosis Capability of Addiction and Mental Health Treatment Services: Implementation Factors Associated with Program Level Changes." *Journal of Dual Diagnosis* 6 (2010): 237–50.

Hazelden, a national nonprofit organization founded in 1949, helps people reclaim their lives from the disease of addiction. Built on decades of knowledge and experience, Hazelden offers a comprehensive approach to addiction that addresses the full range of patient, family, and professional needs, including treatment and continuing care for youth and adults, research, higher learning, public education and advocacy, and publishing.

A life of recovery is lived "one day at a time." Hazelden publications, both educational and inspirational, support and strengthen lifelong recovery. In 1954, Hazelden published *Twenty-Four Hours a Day,* the first daily meditation book for recovering alcoholics, and Hazelden continues to publish works to inspire and guide individuals in treatment and recovery, and their loved ones. Professionals who work to prevent and treat addiction also turn to Hazelden for evidence-based curricula, informational materials, and videos for use in schools, treatment programs, and correctional programs.

Through published works, Hazelden extends the reach of hope, encouragement, help, and support to individuals, families, and communities affected by addiction and related issues.

For questions about Hazelden publications,
please call **800-328-9000** or visit us online
at **hazelden.org/bookstore.**